Praise for *Slow AF Run Club*

"I wish this book had existed when I was a young fat swimmer.
Martinus has compiled a guide that's thoughtful, practical,
and deeply compassionate. Plus-size athletes and aspiring athletes:
this is the book you've been looking for."

–Aubrey Gordon, *New York Times* bestselling author of
"You Just Need to Lose Weight": And 19 Other Myths About Fat People
and cohost of the *Maintenance Phase* podcast

"Moving outward is an act of courage. Martinus used running
as a way to challenge himself and to show others anything is possible.
He is a great reminder that pace doesn't matter; the finish line
welcomes all that take on the challenge."

–Bart Yasso, Distance Running Hall of Fame

"*Slow AF Run Club* is a great resource for any new runner, bursting with
tons of practical tips and personal experience. Martinus is relatable,
funny, and encouraging and has written an extremely approachable
book that could end up changing your health and quality of life!"

–Caroline Dooner, author of *The F*ck It Diet*

"As someone who has been second-guessed on almost every occasion
when sharing my fitness journey, Martinus delivers everything and
more that us slow runners have been searching for! Martinus is like
that supportive bestie who understands the joys and challenges of
running at your own pace when everyone else around you is screaming
weight-loss suggestions. With practical tips, inspiring stories,
and a beautiful welcoming online community, *Slow AF Run Club*
has helped me rediscover the simple pleasure of running and
connect with like-minded individuals who value inclusivity and
connection over competition."

–Meg Boggs, author of *Fitness for Every Body*

SLOW AF RUN CLUB

The Ultimate Guide for
Anyone Who Wants to Run

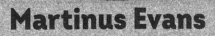

Martinus Evans

AVERY
an imprint of Penguin Random House
New York

AVERY

an imprint of Penguin Random House LLC
penguinrandomhouse.com

Photograph on page iii © Drew Reynolds

Lyrics on page 10: "Send Me, I'll Go," written by Harvey Lee Watkins, Jr., and
performed by The Canton Spirituals; courtesy of East Jackson Publishing Co.

Most Avery books are available at special quantity discounts for bulk purchase for sales
promotions, premiums, fundraising, and educational needs. Special books or book excerpts
also can be created to fit specific needs. For details, write
SpecialMarkets@penguinrandomhouse.com.

LIBRARY OF CONGRESS CATALOGING-IN-PUBLICATION DATA

Names: Evans, Martinus, author.
Title: Slow AF run club: the ultimate guide for anyone who wants to run / Martinus Evans.
Description: New York, N.Y.: Avery, an imprint of Penguin Random House, [2023] |
Includes bibliographical references and index.
Identifiers: LCCN 2022049756 (print) | LCCN 2022049757 (ebook) |
ISBN 9780593421727 (trade paperback) | ISBN 9780593421734 (epub)
Subjects: LCSH: Running—Handbooks, manuals, etc. |
Runners (Sports)—Handbooks, manuals, etc.
Classification: LCC GV1061.E84 2023 (print) | LCC GV1061 (ebook) |
DDC 796.42—dc23/eng/20221114
LC record available at https://lccn.loc.gov/2022049756
LC ebook record available at https://lccn.loc.gov/2022049757

Printed in the United States of America
4th Printing

Book design by Patrice Sheridan

This book is dedicated to the amazing members of the Slow AF Run Club and to anybody who has felt they are too fat, too slow, too old, or too (fill in the blank) to become a runner. This one is for you.

CONTENTS

Introduction   *ix*

Chapter 1
You vs. Your Mind vs. Everybody   1

Chapter 2
Running Slow AF   22

Chapter 3
Shifting to High Gear (aka Running Drip)   35

Chapter 4
Carbs Are Good, F*ck Diets, and Other Running Nutrition   56

Chapter 5
Train the F*ck Up   77

Chapter 6
Boss Up and Get That Race Medal   112

Chapter 7
Recovery Matters   133

Chapter 8
Cross-Train or Die! (Or Risk Injury)   147

Chapter 9
Goals for Days (and Months and Years)   178

Chapter 10
(Running) Communities: Finding Your People   199

Afterword   *215*

Slow AF Run Club Bonus Companion Course   *217*

Shout-Outs and Acknowledgments   *219*

Notes   *223*

Resources   *225*

Index   *227*

INTRODUCTION

"Mr. Evans, you're fat. You have two options: lose weight or die."

It was 2012. I was sitting in my doctor's office, in my 360-plus-pound body. I was fed up with the world telling me all the ways that I was wrong. Getting this fatphobic *bullshit* from my doctor was the last straw. I was hurt, sitting there with my arms crossed, with a tight-lipped smile plastered on my face. While I furiously tapped my right heel on the ground, something else was brewing inside me, as well—defiant anger. A wave of all my experiences of fatphobia rushed over me at once. From being bullied to being forced to shop in the "husky" section while I was growing up to being called names (who could forget being called "tittie boy"?), not to mention all of the laughing and pointing and all of the times that I fought back . . .

"Screw you," I said with a half-cocked smile. "I'm gonna run a marathon." Those seven words changed my life. Something switched on, even as the doctor laughed at me and said that was the stupidest thing he had ever heard in all his years of practicing medicine. Eyes open wide and head cocked to the side, I nodded emphatically as I sucked my teeth and angrily curled my lip. I was using every bit of effort to prevent myself from lunging at him, picking him up by his shirt collar, and tossing him against the wall like a balled-up piece of paper.

"If you run a marathon, you're going to die." Lose weight *or* die. Run a marathon *and* die. Let's just say I left that appointment looking for option C.

I bought running shoes and climbed onto a treadmill that same day. That was the beginning of my journey.

Since then I've run more than eight marathons and more than a hundred other distances in my 300-plus-pound body. I created the Slow AF Run Club and coached hundreds of other runners. I became a global ambassador for a major athletic company, and I've also been featured on the cover of *Runner's World* magazine.

My journey has been far from traditional, and it hasn't been easy. I ran mostly alone and braved just about everything out there on the open road. I've been heckled by people in cars and on bikes, and I've even been harassed by race spectators. People have stopped me countless times to inquire how much weight I've lost (it's none of their damn business, plus this isn't a weight-loss journey). Friends and family have asked me why I participate in "white people sports." I've participated in races where I've come in DFL (dead fucking last). I've run races in which I got lost because they started taking the route signs down. I've run races where they've run out of water and finisher medals, unprepared for the slower runners at the back of the pack. I've written an open letter on behalf of those at the back of the pack, and the response was "Lose weight and get faster."

When I began my now more than ten-years-and-running journey, all I wanted was someone to talk to who had experienced exactly what I was going through. Someone to push back against the stigma and doubt, to put a hand on my shoulder and tell me I was going in the right direction. Now, having learned all my lessons the hard way, I'm ready to share my knowledge and be that voice for the next generation of runners. (Yes, I'm talking to you, the person holding this book!) Runners who aren't running to win, but to celebrate their bodies. Runners who run because they *can*. Runners who have been told that they can't because they look a certain way. Runners in the back who have been forgotten about and left to fend for themselves. It's been a long time coming for us in the back of the pack, but change is coming and I've got your back.

The good news is that the recent cultural shift toward wellness and body acceptance/body neutrality/body positivity is empowering more people of all ages, sizes, and motivations to lace up their sneakers and give running a try.

The bad news? Nontraditional runners in larger bodies are extremely underserved when it comes to resources tailor-made for us. Most instructional books about running are written by elite athletes and former Olympians. They provide advice and plans that are useless for the fat,[1] plus-size, slow, or whatever-you-wanna-call-yourself runners. People like me. The same goes for runners who are beginners, disabled, or dealing with any kind of physical issue that slows them down.

Let's face it: an elite marathoner or an Olympic runner can't and won't give tips about how to prevent brutal thigh chafe or provide running plans for those of us who run 18-minute miles. We are both just like any other runner out there and also completely different. We need specific advice, training plans, and strategies. We need encouragement in a world that has traditionally excluded us at best and bullied us at worst. We need role models.

When I walked out of my doctor's office more than ten years ago, I had no idea that I was on the road to being a role model. Hell, I don't even know if I am a role model or just some guy weighing over 300 pounds and running with goals. My current goal? Help you get moving

---

[1] A word about using the F-word. I'm talking about *fat*! I want you to know that I mean it plain and simple, but it's not for everyone and that's okay. I mean it as a value-neutral description, like describing someone who is wearing a yellow shirt. This is not a license to walk around calling other folks in larger bodies fat. Everyone has their own feelings about the F-word. This is just my take on it.

in the body you already have. Repeat after me: this is not a weight-loss journey! There are so many benefits to running: it helps you feel good, bond with friends/family/pets, get your steps for the day quickly, sleep better, build strong bones and muscles, improve your cardiovascular health, and boost your mental health. The list goes on and on. Running really has nothing to do with a number on a scale or a time on a stopwatch. And to be perfectly frank, running on its own won't cause you to lose weight. During my training for my more than eight marathons, I did not lose any weight. In fact, I gained weight during some of those training cycles

Whatever your size, age, race, gender, or athletic ability, I wrote this book to guide you. I want it to help you feel seen and empowered. I want this voice—my voice—to be your coach and your running buddy every step of the way. You bring the bravery and the energy, and I'll drop the knowledge. Are you ready?

SLOW AF RUN CLUB

CHAPTER 1

You vs. Your Mind vs. Everybody

Cautionary Tale: Don't Get on the Bus!

As I made it to the entrance of the MacArthur Bridge in Detroit, spectators cheered, clapped, and yelled, "You're almost there!" Eking out a smile, I mouthed a quick thank-you, looking forward to what was coming on the other side of the bridge. Methodically I placed one foot in front of the other, legs feeling like lead, trudging through a mixture of quicksand and peanut butter.

I tried to move forward faster, forcefully blowing air out of my pursed lips, tightness radiating from my jaw to the back of my neck, through my traps and down to my lower back, straight through to my feet. *You got this, Martinus. Move faster.* But no matter how many times I repeated this affirmation to myself, I couldn't muster up the burst of energy I needed to move at the pace I commanded of myself. As I passed by the mile marker, I blurted out, "I'm at mile 19 of my first marathon, and shit is getting real." (Yes, I actually said this out loud. Running a marathon will make you do some bizarre things. Like talking to yourself, not to mention running 26.2 miles.)

I was slowly catching up to a man who had slowed his pace to a walk. Making eye contact with him, I nodded. "You got this, brother! One foot in front of the other. You came too far to stop now."

"I'm done," he responded. Shaking my head, I slowed my pace to talk with him in hopes of giving him the words he needed in order not to throw in the towel. If I'm honest, I also did it to silence the voice inside my own head, which was slowly growing louder in volume, telling me to stop running and give up as well.

We continued to run and talk for a few moments, but this guy was burned out. "Hey, bro. I appreciate what you're trying to do, but I'm done." Before I could get a word out, he waved down the SAG wagon (support and gear wagon, a support vehicle—usually some type of van or bus—used during running events, designed to hold food and other equipment for participants and to pick up and carry any runners who can no longer run) as it was passing by. He slowly made his way to the bus, where there were three or four people already inside. They rolled away. I was alone again, just me and the pain cave, the point in a workout or competition where the activity seems impossibly difficult.

As I continued to trudge forward, my shoulders slumped, my pace slowed, and a slight feeling of dread combined with a dash of utter exhaustion came upon me. It was something I had never felt before. I could hear the sputter of the SAG wagon approaching me from behind as the voice that I was trying to silence got louder. *Just quit, there's no point in continuing.* As I tried to shake the feeling off, the SAG wagon pulled alongside me at the same speed I was running. As I heard the whining noise of the vehicle's window lowering, beads of sweat started to form on my forehead. I continued to trudge along, my head down. One foot, then the next. The smoky, musty smell of the exhaust flooded my nose and my taste buds with every step that I took. Next to me, the driver cleared his throat to get my attention. Reluctantly I looked up at him. The guy I had been running with was sitting on the passenger side of the vehicle. As soon as we made eye contact, the inner voice I was battling started up again: *Stop running and get on the bus.* The raspy voice of the driver cut through: "Hey, big man! Do you want a ride back to the finish line like your friend over here?" He pointed his thumb to the passenger side. "Hell no!" I responded jokingly. We both laughed. Inside, I was dying to get on that damn bus.

"Well, I'll be back to come get you on the next go-round." Then he rolled up his window and pulled off.

I instantly stopped smiling and laughing. *What the fuck does that mean?* The inner voice responded, *You should have gotten on the bus.*

The struggle continued. I felt utterly exhausted. I wanted to run faster, but I, unlike the SAG wagon, had no gas left. As I continued to run, a battle raged inside me, similar to one of those cartoons in which the character has an angel on one shoulder and a devil on the other. One part of me was saying, *You got this; keep moving until you get to the finish line.* The other said, *Stop running and get on the bus next time it comes by. You aren't going to make it.*

Exhausted, sore, delusional, not sure who to listen to, I was caught in the middle, so I trudged forward. When I got to mile 21, I once again heard the engine of the SAG wagon in the distance. I was literally shaking my head as it pulled alongside me again. The driver rolled down the window and cigarette smoke escaped.

"Big man, I see that you're still out here?" I nodded. "Are you ready to get a ride to the finish line?" I shook my head no. He drove off.

Mile 24. I was deep in the pain cave. I was determined to stay upright and move forward despite the turmoil I was experiencing. As I moved forward, the SAG vehicle returned. I couldn't look at it. I braced myself to hear the voice again.

"Hey, big man, you're starting to slow down. Hop in, I'll take you to the finish line."

I stopped running and looked him straight in the eyes. My heart raced and I was breathing heavily. My internal battle was still raging. He gestured for me to come closer. "Come on, let's go."

I walked toward the bus. One foot in front of the other. I was empty.

I got all the way to the door, I even touched the handle, and then something stopped me. I shook my head and proceeded to start running again.

A guy on a bike pulled alongside me.

"Do you know where you are?"

"The finish line?!" I responded. He chuckled.

"You're at mile 25; keep going."

About half a mile later, the SAG wagon pulled alongside me, the window already rolled down. At this point my tank was empty and I was riding on fumes. The negative self-talk was still going strong. *If you get on the bus, the pain will go away . . . Don't get on the bus! You're almost there.*

"Hey, big man, get in, I'll give you a ride to the—"

I'd had enough. Expending all the mental energy I had left, I cut him off. "Are you serious? I'm almost there! Why would I get in now? Why would you offer such a thing? Leave me the fuck alone!"

"I'm just doing my job. I can't help that you're fat and slow."

I belted out a single laugh. "Are you fucking kidding me?" Fuming, I stood there, my jaw clenched, shooting daggers at him. His comment stung, but I wasn't going to give him the satisfaction by showing him any weakness. My hands tightened into fists, I swallowed my emotions and held back tears as I looked him dead in the eyes. "Leave me. The fuck. Alone." He stared back at me with a blank face. Breathing heavily, I watched him drive off.

What the fuck was that about? I said to myself, shaking my head while letting out a deep sigh. Emotions were spinning uncontrollably inside of me like a tornado trying to force its way out. Again I swallowed my feelings, took a deep breath, wiped the single tear from my eye, and proceeded to start running again.

Every step hurt more than the last. Yet, every single step was bringing me closer to my goal. The frustration, disbelief, and exhaustion began to fade as the low hum of *something more* began to build in its place.

I made a left turn, and I could see the finish line. I saw Char, then my girlfriend and now my wife, and my mother cheering me on. That building hum turned into a roar that pushed me forward as I gave it everything I had and sprinted across the finish line. I'd done it! I was a marathoner!

I hugged Char and my mother and got my medal. I felt like I could literally do anything. I'll never forget that moment, and everything that had come before it, not for as long as I live.

As we were walking to the car, the SAG wagon slowly passed us. I made eye contact with the driver; he nodded at me with a smirk on his face. I glared at him and nodded back. My eyes followed the SAG wagon until it disappeared into the distance.

This is running in a nutshell. Yes, it's putting one foot in front of the other and swinging your arms and breathing as you carry yourself through the world, but it's also about what's going on in your brain. Running is a struggle of the mind. It's literally you versus the thoughts in your head versus *other people's* thoughts of you versus the thoughts in your head about other people's thoughts of you. Still with me? Basically, for runners—especially runners in larger bodies and others who rarely see themselves in magazines—the art of running is conquering your will, your judgments, and other people's judgments. Because let's face it, people be judgin'. Haters are gonna hate. There's always going to be someone telling you to get on the bus.

What do you do when these things happen? When the going gets tough? Do you quit? Do you fight back? Do you run away? Or do you freeze? All of this comes down to your mindset. Your mindset is EVERYTHING. When the chips are down, what makes a runner a runner is more than athletic ability. It's how you *decide* to handle your challenges.

In this chapter, we'll discuss the keys for building an athlete's mindset. I'll also tackle roadblocks that nontraditional runners face that usually cause them to stop running—perception, fear, and motivation. I'll finish up the chapter answering some questions asked by every beginner, nontraditional, slow, or fat runner.

> **A Note Before We Begin:** What do I mean by *nontraditional runners*? Running and fitness in general have a long-standing tradition of being focused on being thin and pretty damn white. Luckily, in this house we break with tradition big-time. So when I say nontraditional, I'm talking to my slow AF runners, runners in larger bodies, runners of color, runners with disabilities, LGBTQ+ runners, adult-onset runners, senior runners, and any combination of those. I'm talking about anyone who ever felt like they were being scoffed at in the street in their athletic gear, who dreaded gym class, or who left a gym workout feeling discouraged, like they didn't belong. Welcome home!

Success in running—and actually in any other sport—is 90 percent mental and 10 percent physical. That is why we're starting a running book talking about mindset instead of getting straight into warm-up stretches and the best type of shoes to buy. (We will get there, I promise!) Anyone can learn the mechanics of running, like form and breathing. However, mindset is the difference between hitting the snooze button and getting a run in. The difference between not getting to the starting line and getting to the finish line. It steers everything we do. Our mindset is really what drives us forward or holds us back in every activity, every engagement, or every challenge.

Running is one big challenge after another. To be a runner, you need to get your mindset in check.

The goal of this chapter is to light a fire under your ass. We're going to get you thinking of yourself in a different way so you can thrive as the runner that you were born to be! I don't care about your size, your speed, or your athletic ability, you are going to start believing today. Buckle up, because you're in for the mindset ride of your life. By the end of this chapter, you are going to think of yourself as a runner, because . . .

You're a Fucking Runner! Yes! You!

I don't care what anyone says—the internet, social media, or magazines. Hell, I don't even care what you say! You're already a runner and I'll prove it to you.

Here's why. The definition of *run* on Merriam-Webster.com is "to go faster than a walk." This definition doesn't say anything about pace, looks, size, fancy gear, or any of the other stuff that people may have told you matters.

As long as your legs are moving faster than when you're walking, then you are running.

Caveat: There are some mechanical differences between walking and running, and some beginners, though they are technically speaking running, go at a slower speed than their walking pace. Perhaps they are managing pain or have not built up their muscles yet.

People got a problem? Point them to *Merriam-Webster.* You don't feel like a real runner? Well, that's why you're here! Listen to me: if you can move your legs to go faster than a walk, then *You. Are. A. RUNNER!* It may look different from what you see in the Olympics, but it's true.

This is part of a rant I go on when I'm talking to new coaching clients. It's also for anyone who tells me they heard or read something that they need to do or be first in order to become a runner. Nah.

You run? You have the *desire* to run? The second you step out the door, you're a runner. Plain and simple.

"But, Martinus, I'm Not a Runner!"

Hold up. Nope. I'm not buying it. I've heard it before, I'll hear it again. It's one of the biggest things that fat, slow, nontraditional runners struggle with: the fact that they don't actually see themselves as runners. Many have been told by the world that they need to change their bodies *first* in order to start running. Even if no one has said this to you outright, it's everywhere in our culture's messaging, from Fitspo (aka Fitspiration, those posts on social media involving a person with a perfect body and quotes about hard work) to billboards and beyond. Fuck that! You can start running in the body you have right now. You've got everything you need. The last piece is self-perception. Is yours holding you back?

We've all got preconceived ideas about ourselves, including judgments. Take a second to think about the ones you might have about yourself and write them in the space provided below.

_____

_____

_____

_____

_____

_____

_____

For example, maybe you think you're too fat or too slow to run. If you believe that about yourself, you're going to approach running with a lack of confidence or not at all. You may think you need to be a certain weight or shape or skin color to be a runner, but that's a *belief*, NOT a fact.

Reality check: You are not your thoughts and emotions. See, your brain is a factory that manufactures emotions and thoughts. Many of us grow up believing we are the things that we think and feel, without questioning our brains.

This shows up in the way we talk. People don't really say, "I think bad thoughts." They say, "I am a bad person." They say, "I feel fat," not "I am not having a good body-image day." They say, "I am sad," not "I am experiencing sadness."

They say, "I'm too fat or too slow to run," instead of "The way I run will look and be different and that's okay." Here's the game changer: **Not everything you think is true, and not everything you feel is real**. Read that again.

When you are in the moment and things are getting tough, it is easy to forget that your thoughts and emotions exist apart from who you truly are. Becoming an athlete requires you to see your thoughts and emotional processes from the outside. That way you can observe them with some distance. Why is this important? It can help you alter your thoughts and your emotional experiences. You can turn negative thoughts into positive ones and losses into wins. It's all about how you perceive things. You decide what to take from what happens around you. This can be a source of strength or weakness; it's up to you to decide which.

You have to train yourself to think differently about how running relates to your identity. Yes, you are going to have to start thinking of yourself as and calling yourself a runner. The first step toward being the runner that you want to be is to take ownership of being a runner and an athlete.

This is *your* journey to go on, not that of your spouse, your friends, your family, or anyone else. It might even be a journey you are embarking on by yourself, without much support from others. That's okay, too. This is all yours, and you need to adopt the "I'll go, if I have to go by myself" mentality. When I was growing up, my mother would play the gospel song "Send Me, I'll Go" by the Canton Spirituals on repeat. She would literally play it everywhere: in the car, at home, doing the dishes, everywhere. I can hear the words as I'm typing this chapter . . .

I'll go, if I have to go by myself

(have to go by myself)

I'll go, if I have to go by myself

(have to go by myself)

If my mother

(don't go)

If my father

(don't go)

If my sister

(don't go)

Nor my brother

(don't go)

I'll go yeah if I have to go by myself

Even though I dreaded hearing this song growing up, now I think it's really catchy! When I started running way back in 2012, I found myself humming it to myself whenever things got hard. I even went so far as to rewrite it to make it an affirmation to get me going. I would sing,

I'll run, if I have to run by myself

(have to run by myself)

I'll run, if I have to run by myself

(have to run by myself)

If my mother

(don't run)

If my father

(don't run)

If my sister

(don't run)

Nor my brother

(don't run)

I'll run, if I have to run by myself

When things got tough, or even when I felt lonely on a run, this song was a reminder that I was taking my destiny in my own hands. And regardless of who would—or in most cases, wouldn't—run with me, I was going to go do it even if that meant I had to do it alone.

While this was a lonely path, one of the benefits of having this mentality is that you start to build a mental toughness about yourself. Doing it alone is initially scary. You might second-guess yourself constantly, but eventually you start to build self-confidence and toughness because you have to rely solely on yourself to lace up, get out the door, and run. You are a badass on a badass journey, got it? Let's get you on your very own hype train.

Changing Your Perceptions: A Slow AF Guide

First, check your perceptions. Do you choose to see the glass as half empty or half full? Do you choose to see your size or speed as the reason you don't or "can't" run? Or do you see yourself as a fat, slow, and/or nontraditional athlete who can celebrate running regardless of the state of your body?

I opt to choose the positive perspective, and if I'm not feeling positive (because who really does all the time?), then I at least choose to keep things neutral. Let's get real for a second: time is not going to wait on any of us. So don't spend the little that you have on this earth choosing negativity, especially about yourself. Life is too short for that shit. Leave that to the naysayers and the haters.

The body that you have today is the body that you have today. You can do only what you can do today. You can't worry about yesterday, ten years ago, or the point at which you were your smallest (or heaviest) in high school. We need to focus only on the present moment. That doesn't mean that it will be the same tomorrow, next week, or next month. You have to work through the guilt, shame, and whatever other feelings you have around this. The adversities that you've been through make you stronger, not weaker. So despite the feelings and voices from the past that might be dragging you down, you need to remember this: everyone has a day zero (or even multiple day zeros) and that doesn't say anything about you morally.

It doesn't matter where you started (or how many times that you started); it's about where you are going. Remember to choose the positive or neutral perspective. For example, if you tried a running program and it didn't work out how you thought it would in your head, that doesn't mean that the experience was a failure. And it definitely doesn't mean that *you* are a failure. Take ownership of the situation, but learn how to problem-solve so that you'll have more success the next time.

How do you do this? Quite simply, you train your brain. The mind is basically like a computer that only you can program. Just as the food we eat determines how efficiently our bodies run, what we think about ourselves determines how well we run. And we have control over these thoughts. Remember, your thoughts and emotions are not facts; they can be reframed. You can literally train your brain (in fact, rewire it!) with positive self-talk and a belief in yourself. I know this might sound like some life-coach woo-woo stuff, but I am living proof that it works.

Here are some strategies that work for me when it comes to keeping my mind in check.

Use Positive Affirmations

It all starts with what you are saying to yourself. Affirmations are phrases repeated out loud or in your head that are often religious, spiritual, or motivational in nature. They're good because there is scientific proof that our brains respond positively whenever we tell ourselves something new (that is, if the affirmation feels true). So every time I'm having trouble getting out of bed or finding the motivation to do my workout, I recite a positive affirmation and believe it. Trust me, every time I do this, I feel better, and it makes running so much easier.

Here are some of my favorite affirmations:

- No struggle, no progress
- I'll run if I have to run by myself
- I got this!
- Every day I'm shuffling
- Your race, your pace
- You can do hard things
- Slow but show
- One step at a time
- Stay in the moment
- I love hills!!!
- Inclines equal declines

Here are some favorite affirmations from the members of Slow AF Run Club:

- One mile at a time, one step at a time
- Keep going—you never know who you might be inspiring today
- Bad bitches don't stop!
- Focus on the mile you're in!
- This is hard, but I can do hard things!
- The mind gives up long before the body needs to
- Still not dead. Getting stronger with each step!
- Comparison is the thief of joy
- Slow is steady, steady is fast
- Settle in. Hunker down. Chill out.
- I am, I can, I will, I do
- Sexy, sexy, sexy, pace

Use the blanks below to create your own affirmations:

_____

_____

_____

_____

_____

_____

_____

_____

You can also use affirmations to counteract negative thoughts. The next time you notice a negative thought about your running process or body, counter it with an affirmation! Which brings me to my next point . . .

Check Your Self-Talk

Do you say things like "I could never do that," "I'm too fat to do XYZ," "He is so much faster than me," or "She is light-years ahead of where I am right now"? Whoa, whoa, *whoa*! Who the fuck are you talking to? I know you are not talking to yourself that way! Everyone has an inner critic inside them that eats away at their confidence, finds fault and excuses, and creates negativity. Most of the time we don't even consciously notice that this is going on.

Think about where these kinds of thoughts come from and ask yourself whether they are serving you. What might happen if you stopped calling yourself names or using words like *I can't*? How would your life change? Just by taking a moment to notice your own self-talk, you can start catching yourself when you are being negative.

Sometimes you may need a little more help with this. For me, it took years of therapy to learn how to catch and unpack the things my inner critic was saying. When I finally started doing this, though, it changed everything.

An exercise that I found very useful was to give my inner critic a name, a voice, and a personality that makes it quickly identifiable. My inner critic's name is Otis, and he has an old, raspy voice. Think of a drunk uncle, one who be saying random ignorant stuff. Yeah, that's Otis. Sometimes I write down what Otis is saying and repeat it out loud in his voice so I can see how ridiculous the things he's saying are and how they don't make sense.

Sometimes I even have conversations with him and let him know that I'm not here for the BS today and what he is saying is not useful to the cause. I am constantly challenging Otis to move his mindset from one of negativity to one of growth and possibility.

Maybe this sounds a little strange, but it really does work if you put it into practice. The bad news is that your inner critic will never go away; it's inextricably a part of you. However, with this exercise you can work on making its voice less powerful, less of a stumbling block to your achievement. You can separate yourself from that voice holding you back.

Use the space below to name your own Otis.

_____

_____

_____

_____

Practice Delusional Self-Belief

Everything is unrealistic until it's not. Delusional self-belief is just that: believing in yourself no matter what because you know, deep down, it can be true. Think of all the modern technologies that we take for granted. People told the inventors that they were out of their minds until the inventions actually worked. Think of the telephone or aircraft. More recently, naysayers maintained a sub-2-hour marathon was impossible until Eliud Kipchoge did it.

Think about the people who created and accomplished these things. Others thought they were delusional, but they continued to follow through until their ideas came to fruition. If they can do that, why can't you employ some delusional self-belief to go after your dreams?

Hell, if it wasn't for my delusional self-belief, you wouldn't be reading this book. When my doctor told me I was stupid for saying I was going run a marathon, I still went to a running store and bought shoes. That's delusional. I tried and failed multiple times but believed that I would eventually be where I wanted to be.

Look at me now. At the time of writing this book, I have more than eight marathons under my belt and a hundred other distances completed. I've created the Slow AF Run Club, which has thousands of members, and I was on the cover of *Runner's World*. All of this was unrealistic until it wasn't. This is the type of self-belief I want you to have for yourself. Even if you don't believe in yourself now, be delusional and believe in yourself anyway. Sometimes you have to be delusional to even start, let alone to keep going. You have to be the first person who thinks that you're going to achieve what you've set out to do. If you're not sure what that is, try to make a list. Write down a couple of "moonshots." I dare you!

_____

_____

_____

_____

_____

FEAR: False Evidence Appearing Real

Fear isn't real. Most of the things we're afraid of are just products of our imaginations, anxieties about the future. They are concerns and worries about things that don't currently and might not ever exist. Don't get me wrong: danger can be very real. But when it comes to running, how you handle your fear is a choice. What are you afraid of when it comes to running? Looking stupid? Coming in last? Getting swept off the course?

How are these fears and anxieties holding you back?

Take it from me: I've finished last during races, I've been pulled off courses for being too slow, and I'm here to tell you that nobody died, the world didn't end, and I was able to continue to run races. This stuff doesn't make you less of an athlete. In fact, it makes you *more* of an athlete because you didn't quit.

Fear doesn't discriminate between any of us. Hell, I'm afraid that one of these big-ass rats in New York City is going to jump out and attack me during a run. But in all seriousness, I was afraid to call myself a runner when I first started because I was so slow. Even the greats are fearful and lack confidence or have inadequate perceptions of themselves at some point. We're all human at the end of the day. So how do you overcome this roadblock?

Do It Afraid

Seems pretty simple, but looking your fear in the eye and doing what you want to do anyway is huge. Why? Doing scary things gives you grit. It means you become battle tested and do more things that scare you, which will result in more grit, which will result in your becoming the runner that you want to be. Think of it as a fear piggy bank. Every time you face a fear, it's like you are depositing a token into your fear piggy bank. Go out on your first run even though you're afraid? Add it to the fear piggy bank. Call yourself a runner even though you may not feel like one? Add it to the fear piggy bank. Make enough deposits and you can crush your goals all the way to the bank—or the finish line.

Fear Activity

Write down all the things that scare you about running. Get 'em out. If you want, take some time to reflect on these fears. Write down one positive thing that could still come from facing that fear.

Example: I'm afraid of coming in last. ➤ I went to the race, and I finished. I am an example for people who might be afraid to try running.

_____

_____

_____

_____

_____

_____

Mindfulness Is the Key

Because fear is based on what might happen in the future, one way to help fight it is with mindfulness. This means grounding yourself physically and mentally in the moment. There are lots of meditations and mindfulness resources out there, and I'll provide a few below. You can do these anytime: before a workout to center yourself, after a workout to calm down, whenever the going gets tough during a run. Whenever I am fearful or anxious or feel overwhelmed, I like to touch base with myself. Below you'll find my favorite mindfulness activities to keep me grounded. Trust me: this is some pro-athlete shit.

Mindfulness Activities

Tense and Release: Lie down or sit in a comfortable place with your eyes closed. Focus on inhaling deeply for 5 seconds and exhaling for 10 seconds. Repeat until you're calm. Next, curl, clench, or tense your toes as hard as you can for 5 to 10 seconds, then release. Move up your body, clenching and holding each muscle group for 10 seconds: legs, hands, torso, shoulders, even the muscles of your face. Relax and repeat. This exercise is helpful because it brings your awareness to your body in the here and now. It focuses your attention on your muscles and makes you aware that you are strong, powerful, and capable exactly as you are right now. It also provides a sense of control when you feel like you might not have much.

The 5-4-3-2-1 Grounding Technique: I like this technique because I can do it while I'm actually running.

1. Look around you and name **5** things you can see. For instance, a light pole, a stop sign, a person walking a dog, a car, a big-ass rat you're terrified of (shout-out to my New York City runners!).

2. Focus on **4** things that you can feel. Suppose that you notice the ground beneath you, the tightness of your shoelaces, the feeling of the sun on your skin, or a nice breeze. It can be helpful to say these things out loud, if you've got the breath to do it.

3. Name **3** things that you can hear around you. For example, a lawn mower in the distance, the traffic in the background, and kids playing in the yard.

4. Notice **2** things that you can smell around you right now. Is it the smell of grass or perhaps the smell of trash? If you can't smell anything around you, then name two or three smells that you like, such as fresh-baked bread or a flower.

5. Focus on **1** thing that you can taste. You can do this by running your tongue around your teeth and mouth. Do you taste lingering coffee, tea, or candy? Sports drink? Trail mix? If you can't taste anything, then name a taste that you like. There's something about doing this exercise during a run that calms me down and grounds me in the here and now.

Finding an Enemy

Maybe self-talk and mindfulness aren't enough to get you into your running shoes and out the door. Hey, we all may need something different to get us going—even the greats. If ESPN's *The Last Dance* documentary taught us anything about Michael Jordan, it's that he was powered by proving others wrong, so much that it became a whole meme. (And I quote: "That was all I needed!") He had this knack of finding the smallest thing to activate his greatness, whether it was a look from an opposing coach or a pizza. Yeah, a pizza. (Legend has it that Michael Jordan ate an entire pizza himself the night before Game 5 of the 1997 NBA Finals, got food poisoning, and still put up 38 points on the Utah Jazz.)

If you find yourself dragged back by the negativity of others, be like Mike! Keep yourself motivated with an antagonist (or Otis) and use that to power you. There's something about having that inner switch to turn on your competitiveness to rise to the occasion. Show 'em you don't care, even if it's by caring about the work you put in. Somebody said you can't? Do it anyway. Just remember at the end of the day that your biggest competition in running is yourself.

When you call yourself a runner and master your fears, you're on your way to your destiny. Is that dramatic as hell? Yes. But it's true, we're making big moves here!

MINDSET QUESTIONS ASKED BY EVERY BEGINNER, NONTRADITIONAL, SLOW, OR FAT RUNNER

---

1. How do I get over the all-or-nothing mindset (i.e., thinking in extremes, seeing myself as either a success or a failure)?

   The key to overcoming this type of thinking is to learn to be realistic and avoid thinking in negative, absolute terms. Running is a journey, not a destination, so you must understand and embrace the idea that setbacks happen. This is key. You can also work on recognizing your strengths and choosing the positive or neutral perspective in situations versus the negative perspective.

2. How do I overcome comparing myself to others and thinking things like *I should be faster, I shouldn't tire so easily, I should be able to run farther*?

Listen to me carefully: **you are in competition only with yourself.** You can't compare your Day 1 to someone else's Day 100. The only thing that you can do is to track your own progress, stay on the journey, and keep going.

3. How do I overcome impostor syndrome (considering myself not really a runner because I don't think I look like one)?

Separate feelings from facts, take note of your accomplishments, and stop comparing your journey to those of other people. If you need more help breaking out of these unhealthy patterns of thinking, talk to a therapist.

4. How do I deal with negative comments from people?

People's opinions of you are not your business. Add it to your list and prove them wrong like Mike.

5. How do I get myself to go out for a run on those days when the weather is not so perfect?

Running is all about doing hard things. When you do hard things like running in not-so-perfect weather, it builds grit and helps you become a better runner. Also, running in the rain can make you feel like a badass.

6. How can I avoid analysis paralysis when starting out?

Just GET OUT AND RUN. We don't have time for fear and hesitation!

Now that your mindset's in check, you're ready to embrace the badass runner you were born to be. From gear to training plans, to nutrition and race selection, we are going deep on running in the upcoming chapters. Let's goooo!

CHAPTER 2

Running Slow AF

Cautionary Tale: My First Run

The doctor's words were playing on repeat in my head: "Mr. Evans, you're fat. You have two options: lose weight or die."

I hadn't gone to see him for a lecture.[1] Back then, I was working a commission sales job at the Men's Wearhouse, which had me on my feet all day. Those hours had turned into hip pain that sent me to the doctor's office. Which was where he dropped the F-word on me. *Fat. Lose weight or die.*

Angry and defiant, I had responded with a few words that would change my life forever. But you knew that. You read the introduction, right? We've done this part.

"Screw you. I'm gonna run a marathon."

"That's the stupidest thing I've heard in all my years practicing medicine. If you run a marathon, you'll die."

---

[1] Many people in larger bodies often get lectures at the doctor's office. You may go in for, say, a cut on your hand, and the doctor will heckle you about your weight. What does how many stitches I need have to do with my size? I see you, fatphobia.

I wasn't stupid. I was getting a master's degree in health promotion. What I *was* was stubborn. I bought a new pair of running shoes on my way home from that appointment. I was going to run a marathon that same day and prove the doctor wrong.

The fitness center in my apartment building smelled of sweat. The air was filled with the rhythmic pounding of the runners at the back, speeding on the treadmills at what sounded like 100 miles an hour. As I approached, a lump started to form in my throat. What the hell was I getting myself into?

There were three treadmills, and the only empty one was right in the middle, inconveniently sandwiched between two people running like gazelles on the Serengeti.

I got on the treadmill and straddled the belt, sizing up the runners on either side of me. Both looked like they could have been cover models for *Runner's World* magazine. White, thin, wearing short shorts, with long legs that seemed to move effortlessly on the treadmill. Meanwhile, I was 300-plus pounds and Black, and I was wearing long basketball shorts and a hoodie.

I steeled myself. I knew I could do it . . . I just didn't know how. I didn't even know what speed to start the treadmill on. I peeked at the gazelle runners. One had his treadmill set to 10; the other had hers on 9.5. I pressed the speed arrow until it reached 7.

As I watched the belt speed up in front of me, the doctor's words ran on a loop in my head. I would show him how wrong he was about me.

I stepped onto the belt and instantly couldn't breathe. Eternity stretched out in front of me. I didn't know if I was running too fast or too slow. Was the treadmill rejecting my body, or was it the other way around? My calves were on fire. I had to slow down. I reached to turn down the speed of the treadmill but hesitated. I had something to prove, right?

WHAM! Suddenly my legs were no longer under me. Time stopped. My shoulder hit the moving belt. The noise that my body made echoed through the fitness center.

I got up quickly, hoping no one would acknowledge what had just happened.

"Hey, bro, are you okay?" the guy running next to me asked.

"Yeah, I just lost my balance," I said, holding back tears and eking out a smile. I reached up and got my cell phone out of the cup holder. The red timer on the dashboard of the treadmill read *15 seconds*. I was a long way from any marathon.

As I left the fitness center, the thuds of the other runners on the treadmill hit me in the back. I walked home, tears running down my cheeks.

When I reached for the doorknob to get into my apartment, that's when I saw it. *No Struggle. No Progress*, tattooed on my right wrist—a reference to a famous 1857 speech by Frederick Douglass. That was it. That was my beginning.

The start of your running story is probably different from mine. Maybe you tried running in the past and quit because you didn't see immediate progress. Maybe someone told you that you needed to lose weight before you got started. Maybe you haven't started yet because you're afraid of being ridiculed. Maybe you're holding the beginning of your running journey in your hands right now.

Whether you got started and you're looking to jump back in or you've never run a step in your life, take it from someone whose first run was 15 seconds on a treadmill and now has run more than a hundred races and eight marathons. Yes! You can be a runner. PERIOD! It may look different from what you see at the Olympics, but running slow AF is running. I'm here to provide you all the tips, tricks, and lessons that I learned the hard way.

Running 101: Getting Started

First things first! Let's review what we learned in chapter 1! Say it with me: YOU. ARE. A. RUNNER. You were born knowing how to run. It's in you. You know everything you need to know, and at the same time, you also don't know jack. That's why I'm writing this book and why you're reading it. Right? In this chapter, I'm going to teach you how to run. I have trained hundreds of people who start off saying they "couldn't ever." But they can. And you can, too. Here's what I wish I had known before that fateful day on the treadmill. Are you ready?

Running Form

The way you learn to run isn't by running at all. Whether you're running 4-minute miles or 20-minute ones, it all starts with form. Form is the way we hold and move our bodies while we're running. An efficient running form ensures that every movement helps us move forward and doesn't waste energy with unnecessary motion. It also prevents injury. *Fact:* Everyone is different. There's no *perfect running form* for everyone, and your running form will look different from your walking form. (Rule number one of running: Never compare yourself to others. I'm going to say this over and over, so start believing it now.)

Still, there are a few basics to keep in mind. So what are the components of good running form?

Two Mechanisms of Proper Form: The Lean and the Landing

The two components of proper form are upper body posture and foot strike, the way your feet hit the ground as you run. We call this the *lean* and the *landing*.

The Lean

Let's experience a little *lean*. Stand up straight, *proud and tall*. Next, bend your elbows (as if you're running) and pull them back. Tilt your chest forward ever so slightly, as if you're giving a chest bump to someone. Your weight should shift to your toes, and you'll feel like you're falling forward. This is what we call the *lean*, and it's the feeling that you're looking for when you're running. This component of form is important because it keeps the diaphragm open, and as a result, you can breathe more efficiently while running. Also keep your chin up, so that your trachea and throat also stay open, which allows you to breathe more easily and relax, so you can really flow with your stride. No sweat, right?

The Landing

Now that you've gotten the lean, let's work on the *landing*. That's how your feet strike the ground as you run.

The key to maximizing this part of optimal running form is to focus on making sure your feet land right below you. Your legs should only move up and down, like you're marching. Focus on short, quick strides. Most people are tempted to make their stride as long as possible, thinking it'll make them go faster. "Martinus," I hear you saying, "I have watched Usain Bolt crush it in the Olympics, and he is striding OUT." But this is an optical illusion. Even though it looks like professional runners are extending their legs far ahead of themselves, by the time they stride out and land, everything is aligned below them. Keep your legs underneath you.

A Note About Foot Strike: Many books say you should aim for a forefoot (the front of your foot) and midfoot (the middle of your foot) strike without showing or telling you the mechanics of how to get there. The truth is forefoot and midfoot striking are a by-product of landing with your weight below you. If the heel is in line to hit first, but your weight lands on your midfoot or forefoot, you are fine. Focusing on landing under your body makes everything align, which lessens the impact on your joints and just generally feels better all around. It can also help eliminate shin splints, which frequently come from a heavy heel landing.

Putting It All Together

Let's try this out. That's right. We're going to run. Jog in place and make sure your feet land directly below you. Then apply the lean until it drives you forward. Voilà, you're running!

Your Running Form Checklist

Remember that walking form looks different from running form, and what works for you will be different from what works for someone else. Here's a quick checklist for perfect running form:

O Look straight ahead as you run, focusing on a point 6 to 10 feet in front of you.
O Relax your shoulders; don't hunch!
O Keep your body loose as you move.
O Bend your elbows at 90 degrees as you swing your arms.
O Hold your hands loose but not open. (Visualize holding a pebble in your hand. You want that pebble to move freely but not fall out of your hand.)
O Ensure your feet are landing under your body.
O Remember your form is unique to you!

Pacing

Pacing is key for beginner runners and elites alike. *Pacing* just means how fast you go when you're running. If you're like me when I first started out, you may think running means going all out, just like the gazelles that I was sandwiched between early in this chapter. While that may be the case if you are trying to run the 100-meter dash, it's definitely not the case for long-distance running. Like me, many new runners don't pace themselves. We set off too fast out of the gate and burn out too quickly. This is also the main reason many people are in awe of runners. You tell a non-runner you went for a run, and they're likely picturing an all-out sprint.

NAH, that is not the way it goes.

From now on, I want you to think of running like war. Yes, I said *war*. What I mean is, running is all about strategy, and to win you need to find the right strategy to be successful. This includes strategy about pacing. In the world of running, there are multiple paces that you can choose from: recovery pace, tempo pace, long-interval (1,000 meters or more) pace, short-interval (100 meters) pace, and the conversation pace (aka Sexy Pace). In this chapter, we will be covering only conversation pace (but the more you run, the more paces you will add to your arsenal). The point here is there are different paces out there that you can run other than "nothing" or "foot on the gas, all out."

Also, each pace is unique to you. So *your* conversation pace may vary from *my* conversation pace, but the main thing is that we all have one. Which goes back to rule number one of running: Never compare yourself to others. (Remember I said I was going to bring that one back up?)

Why Pace Doesn't Matter

That's right, I SAID IT. Right now, as a beginner, you should *forget* about pace. Ignore the number on the treadmill, the GPS watch, and your phone. I know it's hard. Do it anyway. Speed is not the goal. Forget how fast you're going. This is about learning how to manage your energy and monitoring your effort level. Creating a sustainable pace will build a sustainable running practice.

Conversation Pace (aka Sexy Pace)

Conversation pace, or Sexy Pace, basically means running a slower pace. You're still breathing harder than if you are walking, but it shouldn't feel difficult. It's called *conversation pace* because it's the speed at which you're working hard, but you still have enough air to hold a conversation with one of your fellow slow AF running buddies. My alternative term for this is Sexy Pace because it's the pace you'd go if you were running in slow motion on a beach, *Baywatch* style.

This is the recommended pace for 70 to 80 percent of your beginning runs. Right now, we are not worrying about speed, but about consistency. The more you run at a consistent, comfortable pace, the more likely that pace is to increase and the less likely you are to quit and feel defeated.

People always ask what they should run for first, speed or distance. The answer is always go for distance. Get to the distance that you want to run first, and then go back to work on speed. That will help you build consistency.

Breathing

Many runners who are just starting out quickly find themselves out of breath. This usually means that their pace is too fast, but it can also be due to the fact that they are not breathing efficiently while they're on the run.

Chest Breathing vs. Belly Breathing

There are two types of breathing: chest breathing (shallow) and belly breathing (deep). Belly breathing is also called *diaphragmatic breathing*. While you are running, you want to practice belly breathing. This can take some practice. Here's a short drill you can use to practice belly breathing.

Belly Breathing Drill

1. Lie down on the floor or sofa and place your hands or a light book on your stomach.
2. Breathe in through your nose. You should be able to clearly see or feel your hand or the book rise when you breathe in.
3. Exhale from your mouth, focusing on exhaling all the air out of your lungs. You should see your hands or the book fall. Each

breath out the mouth should take two or three times as long as the inhalation.

With a little practice, belly breathing will become automatic and feel completely natural.

Nose Breathing or Mouth Breathing?
Your goal when running is to take in as much oxygen as possible and expel carbon dioxide as efficiently as you can. As the intensity of your running increases, you'll see that you can't get enough oxygen by simply breathing through your nose, so it makes sense to breathe through your mouth. Many people argue that when you breathe in through your nose, the air that is coming in is being filtered by your nose hairs. However, when you're breathing hard while running, your body doesn't care if you are breathing through your nose or mouth. It's best for you to figure out what's comfortable for you, and do what feels natural. You'll find that the more you run, the easier it is to breathe!

The RPE Scale

Feeling	RPE	Talking ability	Description	Training run
😴	0	Conversation	Feels like sleeping or watching TV.	No effort
😆	1-2	Conversation	Feels like you can maintain for hours. Easy to breathe and carry a conversation.	Recovery
😄	3-4	Conversation	Breathing heavily, can still hold a conversation. Still somewhat comfortable but becoming noticeably more challenging.	Easy
😏	5-6	Sentences	Borderline uncomfortable. Short of breath, can speak a sentence.	Tempo

Feeling	RPE	Talking ability	Description	Training run
😳	7-8	A couple words	Very difficult to maintain running intensity. Speak only a few words and can barely breathe.	Long intervals 1000m intervals
😲	9-10	One word to can't talk	Max effort. Feels almost impossible to keep going. Completely out of breath.	Short intervals 100m intervals

The rate of perceived exertion (RPE) scale is a tool you can use to gauge your effort. This scale ranges from 0 to 10. It's relative for every single runner, and with time, you'll figure out how to work within yours. For most of the runs when you start, you'll be aiming for the sweet spot, an RPE of 3 to 6. You might push yourself to a 7 toward the end of a workout.

Note: A good rule of thumb for every run is to start slow and finish strong. Learning to control your pace and save your energy for the end of your run will give you a much more enjoyable running experience!

Intervals

A strategy that can help you get faster and go farther in your running is called *run/walk intervals*. This form of training is self-explanatory: You do stretches of running broken by stretches of walking, helping you to conserve your energy. You do NOT run until you're exhausted and then catch your breath. (Hell no!)

Choosing Your Intervals

What's the best ratio of running to walking for you? Here are some you might try based on your running experience. Remember, running should feel like a 3–6 on the RPE scale.

Some run/walk ratios for beginners:

- Run 15–60 seconds, then walk 90 seconds.
- Run 15–60 seconds, then walk 60 seconds.
- Run 15–60 seconds, then walk 45 seconds.

You want to set the run interval so you stop before your legs are tired. You should be able to recover during the walk interval and be ready for the next running portion. If you need more of a break, shorten your run interval; don't increase your walk. Our goal is to keep your muscles warm while you're on the move.

> **Pro Tip:** Many devices or apps can help you run intervals. My favorite is a free app called (you guessed it) Intervals. Download it on your phone and get ready to move! GPS watches usually have the intervals function as well.

Your First Run

You know your form. You know how to breathe. You've chosen some intervals to test the waters. There's only one thing left to do: lace up your shoes, get out there, and give it a try.

Here's your plan:

- 5-minute warm-up walk
- 20 minutes of run/walk intervals (remember, you can run as little as you need to)
- 5-minute cooldown walk

Remember how my first run went? I don't want that for you. So always remember rule number one of running: Never compare yourself to others. (I'll repeat this again and again.) I also want you to remember that it's not where you're starting out from, it's where you're going. My journey started with me falling down, and look at me now. Where are you? Where will you go?

I want to congratulate you for having the courage to start. The celebration is in the application. You got this!

Your Running Journal

I would strongly suggest that you start a running journal. A running journal is a great way to track your progress along the way. (It's also a great way to know how many miles you have run in your shoes so you'll know when to replace them. We'll talk about this later.)

Also, if you ever get down on yourself, you can go back and reflect on where you started and see clearly how far you have come. Your training log can be as elaborate or as basic as you want.

Keep your log wherever it suits you—in a notebook, an Instagram account, a blog—and customize it with notes about what matters to you. Running is a great self-experiment! Here are some more factors you can keep track of for each run: weather, fuel, distance, intervals, how your body felt, how your brain felt, how many dogs you saw, and whatever the heck else you want!

RUNNING SLOW AF QUESTIONS ASKED BY EVERY BEGINNER, NONTRADITIONAL, SLOW, OR FAT RUNNER

1. How do I know if my form is right?
   It should feel natural to you and it shouldn't hurt.

2. Should I start timing my pace from my first run?
   No, I wouldn't want to complicate running early on. Instead spend that time getting in tune with your body. Learn what your natural conversation pace is.

3. What if I don't have a dramatic reason to start running?
   That's okay. We'll talk about your "big why" in chapter 9.

4. What do I say to my friends and family members who tell me that slow running isn't running or that intervals don't count as running?

To mind their own fucking business. Your journey isn't their journey.

5. Is there an app to help keep a virtual running journal?

You could use any of the running apps such as Adidas Running, Runkeeper, MapMyRun, Strava, etc. Many of them have space where you can add notes about your run.

I recorded a quick video to demonstrate lean, landing, and breathing. I've also created a helpful sheet you can use to track your training. They're in chapter 2 of your Slow AF Run Club Bonus Companion Course, which you can get access to at slowafrunclub.com/course.

CHAPTER 3

Shifting to High Gear (aka Running Drip)

Cautionary Tale:
The Chafe Monster Is Real (Even Though I Made It Up)

It'd been about three months since I had fallen in the fitness center. I was starting to get the hang of running. I had my headphones on while my feet pounded the pavement. My breathing was somewhat labored, but I didn't feel like I was going to die anymore.

I was taking on my longest run to date—a full hour!—and I felt great about it.[1]

Some things had changed for me, but some had stayed the same. I was still wearing an oversize cotton T-shirt to cover up my belly, long basketball shorts, cotton socks, cotton drawers, and sometimes an oversize cotton hoodie. At that point, this was the athletic gear I felt comfortable and safe in when I was running in public. Even if it was 90 degrees, I still covered up.

---

[1] At this point in my running journey, I was still going by "time ran" instead of "miles ran" because the number sounded bigger and better. What sounds better to you? Saying that you ran for 45 minutes or for 2.51 miles?

As I ran, I started to feel euphoric. A sense of ecstasy, inner clarity, and serenity washed through me. The run began to feel somewhat effortless. Was this the elusive runner's high that I had read about?

Before I could ruminate on this any further, the sensation was ruined by something else battling for my attention: my damn drawers riding up my leg. This had happened to me before while running. Every so often my shorts would ride up my leg. No big deal, right? I'd adjust them during my walking interval and keep moving.

This time it was different. Because I was running longer than ever before, I was getting sweatier than ever. My cotton gear began to hold water like a sponge. I went from having a smooth stride to needing to do a weird leg shimmy every three or four steps to get my drawers to fall back into place.

At the same time, my legs were rubbing and slapping together, producing enough heat and friction to start a forest fire. By the time I finished running, I was sweat-soaked and soggy.

As I got undressed for my shower I noticed that my underarms, my nipples, the space between my legs, and some other TMI crevices were raw and red. I didn't care; everything was going to be okay. After all, I had tasted my first runner's high, and I was going to take a nice hot shower and eat something good afterward.

I stepped into the shower. Big mistake.

The instant the water hit my nipples I yelled in pain. They felt like someone had rubbed them with sandpaper. Instantly I turned my back to the water. Then the stream ran into my armpits, and I banged into the shower door as I tried to escape. The pain felt like someone had poured gasoline on me and lit a match. I'm talking about fire everywhere.

In a hurry to finish up, I grabbed my washcloth, adding soap. When the combination of the soap and hot water hit the crack of my ass, I almost knocked the shower door off of the hinges. I caused such a commotion that Char burst into the bathroom.

"Are you all right in there?"

"It got me!" I responded.

"What?! What got you?" She stepped closer to the shower door.

"The Chafe Monster. I'm on fire everywhere!" I responded.

"Who?"

"The Chafe Monster! I made it up, but it got me!"

She laughed and closed the bathroom door. The lesson here? Don't get caught by the Chafe Monster.

After that day, I knew that I had to rethink my running gear.

Many new runners start out wearing whatever they have lying around the house. Nine times out of ten it's an old cotton T-shirt and shorts. That will cover you for the first couple of runs, but as you start to run more frequently, you'll need to upgrade to something more high-tech.

The right gear can keep the Chafe Monster away, but it can also help prevent injury, make your running more efficient, and even possibly save your life. In this chapter we'll tackle what you need in a basic running kit, why proper gear is important, where to find gear for plus-size runners, and more. Are you ready? Let's go!

Checklist of Gear You Actually Need

Here's a quick list of what you'll need in your basic beginner's running kit. It helps to have enough of each of the clothing items so you can complete three runs a week without having to do laundry.

O Workout clothes made of technical fabric:
      Shorts and pants/leggings (compression optional; more
      on this later)

Shirts (compression optional)

Athletic socks

Hat

O Running shoes

O Hair tie for those of you with long hair

O Sweatproof sport sunscreen (protect your skin!)

O A medium- or high-impact sports bra

O Period-proof running shorts or leggings for that time
of the month, if that suits you better than tampons and/
or pads

Checklist of Gear That Might Be Nice to Have

Here's a list of nonessentials you may want to add to your running kit over time. These can improve your running, but they will cost extra beyond the basics. Think of this as a list of items you might want to invest in over time as you get more serious about the sport. (Psst! Many of these make great gifts OR they are nice rewards to buy yourself after a big race!)

O Running watch/fitness tracker

O Water bottle/hydration pack

O Gloves (depending on the weather)

O Foot and wrist lights (for evening or early-morning running)

O Sunglasses

O A running belt to hold your water, keys, etc.

O LED light vest

About Technical Workout Clothes

When it comes to running, cotton is not your friend (unless you want a visit from the Chafe Monster). That is why you need to invest in some technical running gear. These fabrics keep your body dry and comfortable during your run by wicking moisture away from your skin and to the top layer of the fabric so it can evaporate and reduce friction. Less friction means less chafe!

There are two types of technical fibers: synthetic and natural.

Synthetic Technical Fibers

- **Nylon:** This is one of the most popular fabrics in running wear. It's sweat-wicking, breathable, and super stretchy so it'll move with you for a comfortable ride.
- **Polyester:** This is a plastic-based fabric, which means it's durable, lightweight, breathable, and nonabsorbent. It also repels UV rays and keeps you warm when it's wet, making it ideal for running jackets.
- **Polypropylene:** This fabric is water-resistant, which makes it a great base layer. Regardless of how sweaty you get, it will stay dry next to the skin.
- **Spandex:** Also known by the brand name Lycra, spandex is stretchy and flexible. This synthetic fabric can expand, offering you unrestricted movement, before snapping back and retaining its shape.

A Word About Synthetic Fibers: The negative about synthetic fabrics is that they are made out of plastics and can potentially contribute to plastic waste. However, major brands are starting to make clothes from recycled plastics and clothes meant to be recycled. Also many companies sell pre-owned apparel as well to reduce waste. Nylon was the first synthetic fabric ever produced, and it is made from carbon-based chemicals like those in coal and petroleum. Nylon is not biodegradable and will pollute the planet for hundreds of years. So, what do you do if you want to run green?

Natural Technical Fibers

- **Bamboo:** This is a great eco-friendly alternative to synthetic fibers. It is naturally sweat-wicking, antibacterial, and incredibly soft.
- **Wool:** This ain't Grandma's itchy wool that you grew up with! Merino wool is ideal for both hot and cold weather running, as it is temperature regulating, extremely breathable, sweat-wicking, and antibacterial. It's often combined with synthetic fibers such as spandex to give it a more fitted shape. It's also incredibly lightweight.

Lots of sports brands have their own patented technical material to prevent chafe. Explore which ones have the sizes and cuts you like, but *ditch the cotton*!

Shopping for Running Clothes in a Larger Body

I'm just going to come out and say it: if you're in a larger body, finding workout clothes might be difficult for you.

This is especially true if you're a man (or are looking for masculine-looking workout wear). Rant time: It's a huge letdown to go to the men's section in any store and still see six-pack abs posted all over the place. You see plus-size models and mannequins in many women's sections. WTF? Why the double standard? It doesn't make sense! Plus, if something fits me, I will buy one in every color. **Brands, do you not like money?!**

Women (or those looking to buy feminine workout gear) might have an easier time finding workout gear. The social media revolution of body positivity means that brands often carry plus-size activewear for women right in the store. (I will note that one caveat for this, though, may be sports bras. The difficulty of finding a correctly fitting, supportive bra for people with larger chests, and the resulting physical pain and self-consciousness, can be a huge running deterrent—but they are out there!)

However, if you are a 3XL or larger (no shame in that game, believe me!), don't expect to go into a store and come out with bags and bags full of gear. Don't give up yet, though! I have a few tips and tricks to help you find running gear for every size and budget.

1. **Take your measurements.** This is especially important to do before you shop online. Don't go by size! Since the clothing industry is all over the place with its sizing, I recommend picking up a sewing tape measure. Look for something longer than 60 inches. Write down your measurements. Then while shopping online, you can check sizing charts. This little investment will save you time, money, and heartbreak.

2. **Save the designer running gear until *after* you've run your first race.** It never hurts to invest in a few pieces of workout gear, but don't buy anything expensive until after your first race or big milestone. (What this may be is subjective and thus up to you to determine.) Such an accomplishment shows that you are committed to running and deserve a reward for all the hard work and dedication you put into it!

Where to Shop for Running Gear

Before we get into this, I just want to say up front: NONE of these places are paying me for endorsement. All of these recommendations come from painful experience.

Walmart can be a saving grace. I have lived in many areas in multiple states and Walmart has never failed me for workout clothes. Plus, running gear is often expensive, which can be a barrier for people with a tight budget. So go forth and explore without shame and get something to run in!

Check out Marshalls and TJ Maxx. These two stores can be great—especially if the location has a big and tall section. I've gotten about 80 percent of my name-brand gear from these stores. And here's a big tip: make friends with the employees and find out when they get shipments or ask them to put some things aside for you.

Shop online. Some mainstream apparel companies are making workout gear in more plus sizes now. Check them out with one trick in mind: **look for 90-day free returns.** This is key, because clothing sizes can be all over the place. When I buy running gear, I often have to buy two or three of the same thing in different sizes in order to figure out my size in that particular brand. (Or, as I said before, invest in a measuring tape!)

Try Amazon. If you want to shop at Amazon, just be wary. A 3XL is not always a 3XL, so be sure to check your measurements against the sizing chart! Also, watch out for fitness clothes from the UK and Asia because the sizing will be different from what you are used to.

Notes on Compression Gear

When it comes to battling the Chafe Monster, compression garments are a godsend. Compression gear is a base layer, underwear, or a second skin, usually made of spandex and other synthetic fabrics mentioned earlier in this chapter.

Although there isn't definitive proof, many runners (including me) swear by compression gear and its benefits. These include reduced muscle fatigue, strain prevention, improved perceived exertion, increased power, better jumping ability, better recovery after strenuous exercise, and more. Compression garments are ALSO great at preventing Chafe Monster attacks.

This works in three ways:

1. They hold your flesh—meat, skin, fat, whatever you want to call it—tighter to your body so that it's not bouncing all over the place.
2. They act as a second skin. Compression garments are made with very slick material, so when they rub against each other the amount of friction is relatively low.
3. Since they're made from technical fiber, they also help with drawing moisture away from your skin.

Since adding compression gear to my repertoire, I rarely go on a run or even exercise without some piece of it on. I usually wear compression shorts under my running shorts, and if I'm running for more than an hour, I wear a compression shirt under my shirt. Game. Changing.

Note: You can still get chafe when wearing compression garments. That brings me to my next advice—lube up.

Lube Up for Chafe Prevention

Whether you are large or small, your skin and/or clothes WILL rub against one another while you are running. Without lube to help the ease of movement or protect skin, the Chafe Monster will come visit you. It's only a matter of time.

Below is a list of lubricants that I've personally used to keep the Chafe Monster away. I'm not here to say one is better than the other. We all have different bodies, so experiment and see what works best for you.

- Coconut oil
- Body Glide
- Squirrel's Nut Butter
- Monistat Care Chafing Relief Powder Gel

- Megababe
- Chamois Butt'r

Where to put this lube? Everywhere! In between your rolls and your thighs, under your breasts, in your ass crack, everywhere!!!

Pro Tip: If the lube comes in stick form, I usually buy two of the same stick. I label one stick "Booty" and the other stick "Body." For obvious reasons.

Just remember: When you run for extended periods of time, the lube tends to break down. For me, that generally happens around the 2.5- to 3-hour mark (it may be different for you, but just a heads-up).

I usually put some in my hydration pack to reapply for the days when I'm training for and/or running longer distances like half-marathons and full marathons.

Running Shoes (Yes, You Need New Ones)

Running shoes are the most important piece of running equipment in your arsenal. These are something you don't want to pinch pennies on. *There are no magical shoes that can make running easier for you, but a bad shoe can and will ruin your running.* There's nothing worse than being on a run and having to stop because your shoes are rubbing up against your pinkie toe or because you have a blister.

Furthermore, worn-out or ill-fitting running shoes could cause injury. So if it's been a while since you bought a pair of running shoes, then you guessed it, you need new running shoes!

How to Buy Your First Running Shoes
The only thing that I did correctly on the day of the falling-off-the-treadmill incident was buying new running shoes. It's my infamous

origin story: I was furious about this doctor calling me fat, and I was hell-bent on running a marathon.

As I was driving home from the appointment that would change my life, I passed by a specialty running shoe store. I realized I didn't own a single pair of running shoes, made an illegal U-turn, and headed inside.

At that point I learned how much I didn't know about running or running shoes at all. If this is your first pair or your tenth, you might not know much, either. That's perfectly fine! You don't have to be a shoe expert.

The only thing you need to know is that you need a *gait analysis*. The word *gait* refers to the way you walk or run, including how your other body parts move in relation to your walking and running. Say it loud, say it proud. Say. It. With. Your. Chest. GAIT ANALYSIS!

If you go into a store, say those two words to the staff, and they look confused or respond with "Gait what?," politely excuse yourself and leave! Do not pass Go. Do not collect $200. Do not buy shoes from this place, because nine times out of ten you're not going to leave with what you need.

What Is a Gait Analysis?

A gait analysis (or a shoe fitting—I'll use these interchangeably) is the process by which the store staff will determine which running shoe is best for you.

If you haven't had a gait analysis before, then you're in for a treat! It's one of the greatest displays of customer service that I've experienced.

Here's what you can expect during a gait analysis/shoe fitting session:

- Typically the process takes 20 to 60 minutes (sometimes it is faster!).
- The customer service people will take a foot measurement with a

Brannock Device and then compare the results to the size of the shoes you're currently wearing. Most people need to go a half or whole size larger than their street shoes. You need the extra room to allow your feet to flex and your toes to move forward with each stride.

- They may ask a series of questions about your current running routine, future aspirations, or previous injuries.
- They may check the wear pattern on your current shoes. This can usually tell them what type of gait you have so they can make recommendations based on that.
- They may have you walk around the store or on a treadmill. In this way they can assess your walking patterns, if your arches are collapsing, your ankle mobility, and more.
- They may do the wet foot test (spraying your feet with water and having you step on a piece of paper). This will indicate the type of arch you have.
- They may have you put on a neutral-cushioned running shoe and ask you to run on the treadmill or around the store. Such a shoe has no stabilizing features and thus allows your foot to move and flex without any guidance from it.

Depending on the store that you go to, this may be the most intense kind of shoe shopping you've ever done! After you go through the steps above, the sales associate will bring out a few pairs of shoes for you to try on.

The only way to know how shoes fit on you is to try them on. Be sure to put on both shoes and take them for a run around the shop, on the treadmill, or on the sidewalk. As I said, finding the best fit when you are starting out is very personal. As you get familiar with running shoes, you'll start to develop your own preferences. Also, note that a good running shoe store won't have the same restrictive return policies as a regular shoe store. Yes, they will take your shoes back even if you have run in them outside.

I hear you asking, "Martinus, just how do I know which pair is my solemate?" Here's how to tell if you have the right pair of shoes for you!

When you are standing with both shoes on, make sure you have enough space for your thumb between your longest toe and the tip of the shoe. This will ensure that you have enough room for your toes in the toe box and enough room for when your feet swell.

Next, close your eyes and really FEEL how they are fitting. Imagine running for 45 minutes to an hour. Does anything feel weird, funny, annoying, off, or uncomfortable? I mean any little thing. Maybe the collar is rubbing against your ankle or your pinkie toe is a little cramped.

Those annoyances will be front and center during your run. That cramped pinkie toe is going to sprout a painful blister over time.

If the shoes feel uncomfortable anywhere on your feet, DO NOT BUY THEM! Trust me, your feet will thank you later. **I repeat: Do not buy shoes that are uncomfortable**, regardless of the brand, price, or style of the shoe.

P.S. Don't let the sales associate tell you that they need to be broken in, either. That's a lie. It won't get better over time.

Other Running Shoe Shopping Tips

- The most expensive pair isn't necessarily the right pair for you, so don't be tempted into thinking that a higher price always equals a better shoe.
- Getting shoes at the end of the day helps a lot for proper fit. This is usually when your feet are the most swollen because you've been on your feet all day.
- Ignore any recommendations your friends make. They may have a different running style, gait, and goal than you do.

- Wear the thickest athletic socks you have to try on shoes. This is to ensure they are still comfortable after long runs.
- Shoes that might feel comfortable to you while you are walking around the store won't necessarily feel that way when you are running, so make sure that you always take the shoes you intend to buy onto the treadmill for a test run.

If you're strapped for cash, one way of getting the best of both worlds is going to a store to get a gait analysis and shoe fit, then purchasing your shoes online. You can try to find last year's model of the shoe that they recommend for you for a discount.

Buying Running Shoes Online

I advocate for shopping at your local specialty running store because it helps small businesses and you can also connect there with your local running community. (Most small stores have running clubs!)

At the same time, not everyone has a local running store or the funds to spend there. If you're strapped for funds, buying online is a good option.

When you are shopping online, these are some of the questions you need to ask yourself:

- Are you wearing the right-size shoe?
- Are you an *underpronator*, an *overpronator*, or a *neutral pronator*? (Most runners can run in a neutral shoe, but if your foot tends to roll to the outside or inside of the sole, there are shoes for that!) Don't know what these terms mean? More on this below.
- Where are you planning to run? Do you mostly hit the road or track? Or do you hit the trails and gravel paths?
- Do you want to feel like you're running on a cloud or feel the ground underfoot?

Let's break down why these questions are important and how to address them.

Are You Wearing the Right-Size Shoe?
You need to measure your feet. Did you know that 63 to 72 percent of the population is wearing the wrong-size shoe? Make sure that doesn't include you by measuring your feet before buying running shoes online. You'll need:

- A couple sheets of paper
- A hard, flat surface
- A pen, pencil, or marker
- A ruler or a tape measure

Steps to Measure Your Feet

1. Lay a piece of paper down on a hard floor.
2. While wearing the thickest socks that you typically run in, step on the paper and outline your foot with a pen. (Do this for each foot.)
3. Take the tape measure and measure the length of each foot from heel to longest toe as well as the width (crossways) at the widest point. Yes, include that bunion as well.
4. After measuring both feet, determine your shoe size for different brands by comparing your measurements to their sizing guide.

What If You're Between Sizes?
For running shoes, it's usually best to go up a size. Having a bit more room in the toe box will help prevent black toenails, ingrown toenails, and other foot ailments. Again, it's common for running shoes to be a half size to a full size larger than your everyday shoes. As I said above,

don't assume you know your size. Measure and check your results against the brand's size chart.

Are You an Underpronator, an Overpronator, or a Neutral Pronator? Many runners can wear a neutral shoe, which has no stabilizing features. But no two runners are exactly alike.

If your feet tend to roll out when you run, you might need shoes for underpronation, which is also called *supination*. If your foot rolls inward, you are likely overpronating and need shoes that will stabilize your foot. Here is a helpful chart of the signs for each.

Runner's Gait	How Your Foot Lands When You Run	Wear on the Soles of Your Shoes	Type of Shoe to Buy
Neutral Pronation	Mostly square to the ground— balanced	Wear on the soles is mostly even.	Neutral running shoe
Underpronation (Supination)	Toward the outer edge of your shoe	Wear on the soles is toward the outside of the shoe.	Supportive neutral running shoe
Overpronation	Toward the inner edge of your shoe	Wear on the soles is toward the inside of the shoe.	Stability or motion-control running shoe

If you overpronate or underpronate, there are shoes that can help you.

Where Are You Planning to Do Most of Your Running?
Are you mostly on the local track or road? Or do you hit the trails and gravel paths? You want to choose a shoe that is either road-running or trail-running.

- **Road-running shoes** are best for people who run on sidewalks, roads, treadmills, or a paved or rubber track. The shoes typically have flatter, smoother soles to create a consistent surface for running on paved roads. They are light and flexible and made to cushion or stabilize feet during repetitive strides on hard, even surfaces.

- **Trail-running shoes** are best for people who run off-road routes with rocks, mud, roots, or other obstacles. They're generally stiffer through the midsoles for more support on rugged trails and uneven surfaces. Sometimes they have protective plates underfoot to help shield your feet from rocks or sharp objects. They have bigger lugs or cleats than road-running shoes for better grip on uneven terrain.

Do You Want to Feel Like You're Running on a Cloud or Feel the Ground Underfoot?

It's not a trick question; everyone has different preferences and needs!

If you want to feel like you're running on a cloud, then maximum cushion or maximalist shoes are what you want. They offer thick cushioning in the midsoles to give an ultimate plush feel underfoot. If you're a person of size who is running long distances or participating in multiday races (or all of the above!), the comfort of thicker, softer foam underfoot may be your ally.

Super-soft cushioning isn't for everyone. If that's the case, but you still want some cushioning, then moderately cushioned shoes may be just what the doctor ordered. They strike a balance between pillow-soft comfort and thin or no cushion. You'll likely find a variety of shoes in this category.

If you want to feel more connection between you and the ground, then minimal cushion or barefoot shoes may be for you. People who swear by these types of shoes say they closely mimic a more natural gait and offer the closest feel to being barefoot while running. These shoes typically don't provide any arch support or stability features, so they can be a source of injury to runners, who often have weak glutes and shortened Achilles tendons.

More Tips for Buying Running Shoes Online

Watch and read running shoe reviews. In this day and age, you can pretty much crowdsource everything. Once you find shoes you're thinking of purchasing, do a quick search on YouTube, Google, or whatever the popular search is when you are reading this book to see what the running public is saying about the shoe. My general rule of thumb is to try to find someone of a similar size and body shape to me.

Especially look for feedback on the room in the toe box, the sizing, or any quirks the shoe might have. You'll find that runners usually have strong opinions about their shoes. You just want to do your due diligence before buying the shoe.

Buy from an online store with a 90-day return policy. I said it before and I'll say it again: Find a place with a lax return policy. I'm looking for free 90-day returns with a "no questions asked" return policy. This type of return policy gives you time to live with your new running shoes. If they don't work, you return them for something that may work better for you! Easy.

Buy multiple pairs. This can be useful when you're running consistently AND if you have the funds. Once you find a pair of shoes you love to run in, buy a couple of pairs. (This is especially true if you find they're on sale!)

Shoe companies change their shoe designs every year. Sometimes it's small aesthetic changes; other times it can be full-blown fit and composition. Next year's shoes may come out and you may hate them. I've straight up bought four pairs of the same shoe because I found the right pair for me. If you can, find what you like and stock up. I don't want you to be stuck like chuck. If you do road running *and* trail running, you definitely need both kinds of shoes.

Retiring Your Running Shoes

As a general rule, running shoes should be retired every 300 to 500 miles. But if you have a larger body, you may need to change your shoes every 100 to 300 miles. Keep track of the purchase date in your training log, and record the miles daily so you know when it's time to get a new pair.

Most running apps have a feature that tracks the mileage of your running shoes, too!

Signs You Need to Replace Your Shoes

If you forgot to track your shoe mileage that's okay, too. Some external signs will reveal that it's time to replace them:

- The bottoms or sides are visibly beaten up.
- The treads are worn out.
- The midsole is wrinkling.

Also, pay attention to how your shoes feel over time. If your favorite pair is leaving your legs or feet noticeably tired after each run (and you can't chalk it up to a more intense training plan or another shift in your habits), it may be that the cushioning has lost shock absorption. It's time to retire those puppies.

RUNNING GEAR QUESTIONS ASKED BY EVERY BEGINNER, NONTRADITIONAL, SLOW, OR FAT RUNNER

1. Are shoes really that important?

   Absolutely! Worn-out or ill-fitting running shoes can cause injury. I want you to stay injury-free for as long as possible.

2. **How often should I replace my shoes and gear?**

A general rule of thumb is you should retire your shoes every 300 to 500 miles. If you are a person of size, this can be more like every 100 to 300 miles. Your mileage may vary depending on the brand of shoe, the cushioning, and other factors.

3. **How do I get that smell out of my technical fabrics?**

After a run, rinse them in water and then hang them up to dry before washing. If they're really stinky, add a cup of vinegar to your wash.

4. **Is gait analysis worth it? How much does gait analysis cost?**

Yes! A gait analysis is most definitely worth your time. As for the cost, they are usually free unless you're going to a specialty clinic. So you might as well get one! You've got nothing to lose and everything to gain!

5. **How often should I have my gait analyzed?**

I would say once a season or any time you feel your current shoes are off.

6. **Once I find a shoe I like, should I stick with it?**

If it ain't broke, don't fix it. I know people who have rocked a specific brand and type of shoes for years. But remember shoe designs change from year to year. When you're buying new shoes, try them on even if that particular shoe is your longtime favorite.

7. **How many miles does it take to "break in" a new pair of running shoes?**

First off, they should be comfy from the start. New shoes should fit like a gem when you first get them. Still, I would say it could take 3 to 10 miles to get the factory newness off of them. Your mileage may vary.

8. **Do I need to break in new shoes before a race?**

Listen to me and listen to me good! Don't try anything new on

race day! Nah, nope, uh-uh, we don't do new shoes on race day. I'll
tell you why in chapter 6.

9.   Help, what do I do if the Chafe Monster gets me?

I usually clean the affected areas (including the inside of the
butt cheeks!) with some hydrogen peroxide or witch hazel and
then apply liberal amounts of Vaseline, coconut oil, or A&D
ointment to them!

Ready to Run?

Now that you got your gear and your shoes, you're ready to run. We'll
tackle running nutrition in the next chapter!

CHAPTER 4

Carbs Are Good, F*ck Diets, and Other Running Nutrition

Cautionary Tale: Tree Stump Confessional

I used to feel like I couldn't run a race until I had conquered the distance a couple of times in training. (As it turns out, I was completely wrong about this, but that's for another chapter.) On this particular run day, I was attempting to run my first 10K ever.

I had my running lube slathered everywhere and I was rocking tech fabric. No Chafe Monster was going to hold me down anymore. My water bottles were filled and the weather was perfect for running.

I was in the zone. Moving forward felt effortless and the world couldn't touch me.

A stranger honked a car horn at me and yelled, "Good job, big man!" I wasn't even fazed. I just waved and kept moving.

I made it to the halfway point of my run with ease. There's no other way to say it: your boy was killing it out there! And then out of nowhere, I felt something I'd never felt before. It was like a haze of brain fog, but throughout my whole body. I tried to shake it off and push through. I was only 30 minutes from home.

Just keep moving, I thought to myself as I continued to trudge along.

Just keep moving.

Just. Keep. Moo-ving.

It started to feel as if I were running in a mixture of cement, molasses, and peanut butter. No matter how much my mind was telling my legs to go, they weren't having it. Eventually it became a struggle to even lift my feet off the ground to move forward. That's when I saw a tree stump on the other side of the road. I used the last fumes in my proverbial tank to cross the street. I tried to ease my body onto the stump, but my legs collapsed.

Hanging my head in defeat, I called Char for a ride. During the drive, I stared hopelessly out of the window, trying to figure out what had gone wrong. I wasn't dehydrated and it wasn't heat exhaustion. I had felt amazing until I didn't.

It was like I had just run out of gas.

"Are you hungry? Do you want to stop and get something to eat before we get home?"

"Yes, I'm starving right now."

"Did you eat anything before you left for your run?"

"No, I usually don't . . ." Before I could finish what I was saying, it hit me. I knew that I needed to rethink my running nutrition. The following weekend I ate before attempting to run a 10K again, and I got through it with no issues.

In this chapter I'll provide a simple breakdown of how the body uses food for fuel. I'll talk about how eating to fuel a run and eating for weight loss are two totally different things and why food is CRITICAL to running performance. I'll also include fueling strategies that have worked for me at different running distances.

LEGAL AF DISCLAIMER

I'm not a nutritionist or dietitian, but I have studied anatomy and physiology. I've attended nutrition seminars and courses during the ten years that I've been on this running journey. I'm going to provide some basics in this chapter that should get you started, but remember to take everything in this chapter with a grain of salt. (We'll talk about salt later, too.)

Everything I tell you here is based on what has worked for me personally. Your mileage WILL vary physically and metaphorically. I recommend that you reach out to a sports nutritionist if you want more specific information, meal plans, or professional advice.

Why Running Nutrition Is Important

Running nutrition is critical to running performance. Not paying any attention to it will cause you to hit what runners call the wall. You'll end up on the side of the road like me. Neglecting it could also leave you with stomach issues and unnecessary pit stops. You won't live up to your greatest potential. Proper nutrition simply makes a world of difference in your runs.

Fuel for Thought

Before we talk about strategy, let's talk about the nutrition basics. When it comes to running, food is fuel. It's not about good food versus bad food. It ain't about "clean" food. It's not about weight loss or your appearance. It's about what food can do to optimize your performance and mental state. The right nutrition for you is flexible and is based on what you can access geographically and financially. It's not about what some Instagram influencer is trying to hawk.

By the end of this chapter, you'll have some basic knowledge about nutrition. We'll also counteract some of the brainwashing that diet culture has imposed on all of us. But first, it's time to tune out the noise and get real about the basics.

Running Nutrition Staple #1: Carbs

Carbohydrates Are FUEL and They Are Good for You

Diet-culture brainwashers may have you thinking that you don't need carbs or that you should eliminate them entirely out of your diet. I call bullshit. Simply put: Humans need carbs. Period! However, athletes especially need enough carbs to fuel their active lifestyles. Carbs are the building blocks of energy, meaning they are our body's preferred fuel source. They provide energy to every muscle function in your body whether you are running, sitting, standing, or lying on the couch watching Netflix.

Carbs work well because your body breaks them down into glucose. Glucose, or blood sugar, is the main source of energy for your body's cells, tissues, and organs. Glucose can be used immediately or stored in the liver and muscles for later use.

If your body does not have carbs available to create more glucose, it has to work much harder to access other fuel in the forms of fat and protein—not in a good way. In direr situations, your body will leach energy from your bones and muscles. This is not an efficient way to fuel our runs!

Often people notice that a run can feel much more difficult after a few miles if they don't have enough carbs to get them through. Don't skimp on the carbs. Trust me.

What Are Some Carb-Rich Foods?

High-carb foods come in two forms: sugar or starch. I'm talking table sugar, the sugars of fruits, and the starch in grains and in some veggies such as corn, peas, and potatoes. Fiber is also a carbohydrate, but humans lack the enzyme necessary to break fiber down into a usable fuel source.

Carb-rich foods can be divided mostly into two categories: **complex carbs** and **simple carbs**.

Complex carbs are found in higher-fiber sources. They are called *complex carbs* because our bodies work harder to get past that nondigestible fiber to access the fuel source of carbs. In other words, the process is more complex. Some examples of complex carbs are:

- Whole wheat products
- Steel-cut oatmeal
- Brown rice
- Quinoa
- Fruit
- Peas
- Corn
- Beans
- Potatoes with their skins

When distance runners are competing and training, **simple carbs** are their best friend. Simple carbs are found in foods with little or no fiber. Our bodies break down and digest these foods more easily. The process is simple. Some examples of simple carbs include:

- White grain products like pasta or bread
- White rice
- Potatoes without their skins
- Table sugar (raw sugar, brown sugar)
- Corn syrup and high-fructose corn syrup
- Glucose, fructose, and sucrose
- Fruit juice and fruit juice concentrates
- Candy

- Processed foods such as potato chips, granola bars, and crackers

So . . . What Do You Eat?

It's your personal choice, but in my opinion, no types of carbs should be off the table (unless you have a gluten allergy, but that's another book entirely!). Even for people who aren't physically active, brains require carbs to function properly.

Sometimes complex carbs are most beneficial for fueling our bodies, and other times simple carbs are best. We can choose the right carbs that will help us meet our goals.

Complex carbs are typically most helpful for us to lean on in our regular day-to-day meals, as the fiber lends increased feelings of fullness and satisfaction and helps to regulate blood sugar and bowel movements. It is also important that your pre-run fueling includes some complex carbs, because they are absorbed more slowly into the bloodstream and thus will give your body a steady energy supply for longer.

During a race or training run, simple carbs are ideal because they move easily into the bloodstream to be converted to energy efficiently.

After a run, you can replenish stored carbs with simple carb foods because the body is primed to move those carbs quickly into storage. Then return to your typical daily diet, including complex carb foods.

Running Nutrition Staple #2: Protein

Proteins Are Vital for Organs, Muscles, Skin, Hormones, and Life

Protein is essential to building bones and body tissues, such as muscles. It also participates in practically every function of your organs and cells, playing a part in metabolic reactions, immune responses, and blood sugar regulation, just to name a few things!

Needless to say, our bodies need protein. While they don't

necessarily prefer protein as an energy source, if you don't have enough carbs or stored protein, you'll start breaking down muscle for fuel. That's why it's key to eat adequate protein.

For athletes like you and me, protein builds and repairs your muscles, ligaments, and tendons after a long run or a tough workout. Physical activity creates small tears in your muscles that need to be repaired. If you are consuming an adequate amount of dietary protein (somewhere around 0.5 to 1 gram of protein per pound of body weight each day), your body will repair these small muscle tears easily, building even stronger muscle tissue. In short, GAINS!

What Are Protein-Based Foods?

Luckily for us, lots of foods contain protein! Most animal products have significant amounts of protein in them, including meats, fish, poultry, eggs, and dairy (except butter, which is pure fat). Many plant foods also contain protein, such as whole grains, rice, beans, and even leafy green veggies. Here's a list to get you going:

- Meat such as pork, beef, or game
- Poultry
- Fish and shellfish
- Eggs
- Dairy products such as Greek yogurt or cheese
- Nut butters
- Tofu
- Lentils and beans
- Quinoa
- Whole wheat bread

Complete vs. Incomplete Protein (aka Why We Need Carbs AGAIN)

Proteins fall into two categories: **complete** and **incomplete**.

Complete proteins contain all the essential amino acids (building blocks of protein that our bodies are unable to make from other molecules). This means that our bodies can do more with complete proteins per se when they are digested and absorbed. Most animal products, such as chicken, eggs, dairy, and seafood, are complete proteins made up of all nine essential amino acids, but there are some plant-based complete proteins as well. These include quinoa, buckwheat, and soy.

Incomplete proteins lack one or more essential amino acids, so our bodies are limited in what they can do with these proteins all on their own. In order to get the full benefit of a complete protein, they often need to be consumed with another incomplete protein, usually a carb. This provides all the essential amino acids needed for proper absorption.

Incomplete proteins that we can put together to create complete proteins are called **complementary proteins**.

Nearly all plant proteins are incomplete and need complementary proteins in order for us to get the full benefit of them. Rice and beans, macaroni and cheese, or peanut butter and crackers are all examples of complementary proteins combined with carbs to provide complete proteins.

Running Nutrition Staple #3: Fat

The Notorious F.A.T.

Despite the terrible rap they got in the eighties and nineties, fats play a crucial role in our key bodily functions. Fat protects our organs, helps us absorb important vitamins and nutrients, aids hormone production, and performs other functions. Muscle growth is also dependent on a fat-based steroid hormone. Translation: If you want to build muscle, you need fat!

Although carbohydrates are our prime fuel during physical activity, we still use some fat to keep ourselves going. During lower-intensity and long-duration physical activities, fats can be our primary energy source, although they don't provide quick bursts of energy needed for speed. The more intense the exercise, the less fat and the more carbs our bodies use. The only time we don't use fat as a fuel source is during high-intensity cardio exercise. This means we need fat available for our bodies to use as fuel.

While studies show that metabolic adaptations do occur as a result of high-fat fueling, claims that high-fat, carbohydrate-restricted diets improve performance in competitive athletes have not been proven. Fat is an inefficient fuel, so carbs are still the optimal fuel source for runners. Some sources of fat include:

- Plant oils (olive, canola, flax, coconut)
- Butter or ghee
- Nuts and nut butters
- Oily fish
- Peanuts
- Avocados
- Hummus
- Seeds (pumpkin, sesame, sunflower)

Running Nutrition Staple #4: Water

Take it from me: you've got to hydrate, hydrate, hydrate. When you're running. When you aren't running. It's just a fact.

Water makes up about 60 percent of your body and serves a number of essential functions to keep you going. It regulates your body temperature by sweating and with respiration, lubricates your joints, helps metabolize and transport nutrients like carbs and proteins in the bloodstream throughout your body, helps to flush waste, acts as a shock absorber, and forms saliva. Water is SO important to our lives that we can't survive more than three or four days without it.

When it comes to running, water is important because of the increased risk of dehydration. This is especially true when it's hot out.

We lose water in so many ways. We lose it when we sweat, when we go to the bathroom, and even when we breathe!

According to Randall K. Packer, a professor of biology at George Washington University, under extreme conditions we can lose 1 to 1.5 liters of sweat per hour. That is why it's important to stay hydrated. If you don't replace the water you lose during running or exercising, then your total volume of body fluid could fall at a dangerous rate, and most important, your blood volume may drop.

When you have too little blood circulating in your body, your blood pressure can fall to levels that can be fatal. Also, your body temperature rises when you stop sweating. Dehydration that causes a loss of more than 10 percent of your body weight is a medical emergency, and if it is not reversed, it can lead to death.

I don't want to scare you too much. I just want to provide the facts so that you'll stay hydrated.

Lucky for us, we can get our liquids from sources other than pure water. Some foods provide us with water as well. Furthermore, other fluids such as juice, milk, or sports drinks can also keep your hydration levels up.

Trust me, staying hydrated is worth it.

Putting It All Together

Now that you have the nutrition basics out of the way, let's talk about how to best use them to fuel your body and mind for your runs. In case you skimmed the introduction, **this is your reminder that I'm not a nutritionist or dietitian,** so consult professionals for personalized professional advice. I'm here to share with you what worked for me. The fueling that is best for you may be different.

Running fuel strategy can be broken down into three different stages: pre-run, during the run, and post-run. Each part of the strategy is designed to get you to the finish line victorious.

Before I knew better, I usually didn't eat until after my runs. It was a habit that I picked up because I would run the first thing in the morning. I would just wake up, brush my teeth, and go run. The incident that I described at the beginning of this chapter changed everything.

The strategy below is simple but could help prevent you from crashing. The right food can make you a better runner.

Pre-run Fueling

Pre-run fueling is all about priming and fueling your body for the particular distance you're about to tackle.

> **Short runs, defined as runs shorter than 75 minutes or between 1 and 5 miles at a 15-minute-per-mile pace:** Since our bodies store carbs for up to 75 to 90 minutes of exercise, this type of run is easy. Try having a snack/small meal of simple carbs 30 to 60 minutes prior to your run. Your body will have started digesting the food and you'll have some energy available.

> **Long runs, defined as any run longer than 75 minutes or greater than 5 miles at a 15-minute-per-mile pace, OR performance-intensive days like race day:** Eat a small meal 2 to 3 hours before you go running. Caveat: If waking up early in the morning to eat 2 to 3 hours before your run isn't feasible, make sure to eat a meal that is high in complex carbs and protein the night before. Then have a small meal or snack that morning 30 to 45 minutes before you start running.

Whether it's a short or long run, you should aim for your meals to be high in complex carbs and protein, but low in fat. This is not a rule that's set in stone. In fact, just the opposite: you're going to have to do a little bit of trial and error to see what foods and nutrient combinations work best for you.

Pre-run Food Ideas

- Granola bar and a banana
- Cheese quesadilla on whole grain tortilla
- Apple with nut butter
- Egg on whole grain toast
- Whole grain crackers with cheese or hummus
- Whole grain tortilla and deli meat roll-up
- Peanut butter and jelly sandwich on whole grain bread

Pre-workout drinks are also an option. All the benefits can be obtained with food, but some people do prefer a commercial beverage. Do what works best for you!

Foods to Avoid Immediately Before a Run

- Ribs, brisket, burgers, or other high-fat meals
- Salads
- High-fiber foods

Pre-run Hydration

I aim for 4 to 8 ounces of fluids the night before, and then 10 to 16 ounces of fluids—mostly water—before exercise.

On-the-Run Fueling

Our bodies can store some carbs, but those stores get depleted after 75 to 90 minutes of running.[1] That's why you'll need to consume additional carbs DURING running. Yes, you'll need to literally eat on the run. This is where specialty items like gels, bars, jelly beans, or other foods come into play.

---

[1] This can vary somewhat based on things like individual differences in carb storage, the pace of running, and the difficulty of the terrain.

The goal of fueling during your run is to never allow the tank to get empty, and the only way to do that is to be fueling **before** you start to feel fatigue. I'll repeat it again: **never wait to fuel until you need it, because by then it's too late.**

You should start refueling sometime between 30 and 45 minutes into your run. The general guideline for the carbs a runner needs to consume while running is 100 to 250 calories per hour of running (or 25 to 60 grams of carbs per hour).

That said, a runner's exact fuel needs vary from person to person. As a larger individual, I find that the general guideline doesn't provide enough calories for me. It leaves me a bit hangry (hungry plus angry) during long runs.

I found a calculation that provides me with a more accurate estimate of calories that I need to consume per hour.

> **Trigger Warning:** This calculation strategy isn't ideal for someone trying to avoid calorie counting. If you're in recovery from an eating disorder, trying to skip out on diet culture, or just plain trying to keep things simple, skip this and stick to the general guideline: fuel early and often. Look after yourself. Good? Good.

For those of you who are looking for the exact number, here's the formula I use:

$$0.63 \times [\text{body weight in pounds}] \times [\text{how many miles you run per hour}] \times 0.3$$

Step 1. Determine your running calorie expenditure per mile.
   Multiply 0.63 × your body weight in pounds.
Step 2. Determine your goal race pace or how many miles per hour you'll run.
   Example: A 13-minute miler will cover 4.6 miles per hour.

Step 3. Calculate your hourly expenditure based on your goal race pace.

> *Example: A 13-minute miler would multiply 4.6 by the number they got from step 1.*

Step 4. Determine your hourly calorie replacement needs.

> *Multiply 0.3 × the figure from step 3.*

So for me the calculation comes out to be:

$$(0.63 \times 350 \text{ lb}) \times (4.6) \times (0.3) = 304 \text{ calories per hour}$$

This is about 50 calories an hour more than the general guidelines. If I followed the standard guidelines for a 6-hour marathon, I'd be missing an additional 300 calories that I need. Would those missing calories make me hit the wall? I'm not sure, but I wouldn't want to risk it.

A Special Note About Race Fuels

As far as race fuels, runners typically rely on sports drinks and running fuels such as gels, gummies, and other snacks high in sugar, such as candy bars, gummy bears, and dried fruit. If you want to bring any of these with you on the course (and I recommend you DO to maintain that intake we talked about), you have to test them out before you race.

Experiment, experiment, experiment to find out what works best for you. Let me tell you that there's no way to get around this! Do it during your training runs—repeat after me, **nothing new on race day!** (*This is not going to be the last time I am going to say this to you. You've been warned.*) If you want to try something that you read about, do it during your training runs. It's also the best time to practice timing your intake.

I'll say it one more time for the folks in the back: **do not try a new**

fueling source for the first time on race day. Stick with what you know unless you absolutely cannot. I'll say two words about this: Porta-Potty visits.

On-the-Run Hydration

Hydrating during your run is all about balance. Finding that sweet spot between dehydration and overhydration (hyponatremia) is key, especially when you are training during the summer months. Even being 1 percent dehydrated can affect your performance. Don't rely on your thirst as the gauge to determine when you need to drink. Thirst is usually a sign that you're already dehydrated. (On the flip side, over-hydration can be equally dangerous and even life-threatening. This occurs when the body has too much water and not enough sodium, so it's important to limit your water-only intake and replenish electrolytes by consuming salt-rich foods and sports drinks or adding some type of electrolyte mixture to your water.)

I personally drink 4 to 8 ounces of water or a sports drink every 15 to 20 minutes (sometimes a little more on hotter days). You need to take the time to figure out what works for you. Some sports watches have a drink reminder you can set for specific intervals. Try alternating between water and sports drinks in different combinations. As mentioned above, part of drinking on the run is about replenishing electrolytes, too.

Post-run Fueling

After your run, what you eat and when you consume it determines how your muscles recover. I like to focus on eating something with carbs and protein—specifically a ratio of 3:1 or 4:1 carbohydrates and protein. Research has shown that this ratio has the best effect on recovery. I'll eat this light snack or meal 30 to 60 minutes after finishing my run. (Research has shown that your body is the most primed for nutrients during this period.) Then I will eat again within 2 hours.

Post-run Food Suggestions

- Chocolate milk (don't let the diet culture talk you out of this—chocolate milk slaps)
- Smoothies
- Fruit with nut butter
- Pasta with protein and veggies

A Quick Note on Supplements

Peep this: The global dietary supplements market size was valued at $151.9 billion in 2021, and it's looking to expand at a compound annual growth rate (CAGR) of 8.9 percent. What does this mean? The industry is doing a great job of making a shit ton of people buy dietary supplements. It's a slippery slope when it comes to dietary supplements. While these could be beneficial to those who are deficient in certain vitamins, my question to you is: Do you really need them? Or are you taking them because you saw an ad praising them or a friend is taking them? This is a tricky topic. I'm not going to lie, I take supplements under the direct supervision of my nutritionist and healthcare provider. Those in charge of my medical care schedule me for regular blood tests so I will know if and when it's time to stop taking supplements. Just because supplements are available for you to buy doesn't mean that you need them. Needless to say, talk to a nutritionist or your healthcare provider about what supplements you should or shouldn't take.

Post-run Rehydration

After a run or a workout, rehydration is important as well. There are a couple of ways to know whether you are rehydrating adequately after a workout. The easiest and simplest way is the pee test. Keep drinking water or sports drinks until your urine is a pale yellow color. If you're going a lot, then you're likely drinking enough, too.

There is a more technical formula you can use for this.

> **Trigger Warning:** This next method requires you to weigh yourself multiple times. Skip this section if it's going to bring up any nasty diet-culture feelings or ruin your recovery. Look after yourself, okay?

To get an accurate assessment of my hydration, I use something I call the sweat loss method.

Step 1. Get naked and weigh yourself before your run.
Step 2. After your run, get naked and weigh yourself again.

Your sweat loss is equal to your body weight (pounds) before exercise minus your body weight after exercise. You should drink 20 to 24 ounces of water or sports drink for every pound of weight lost.

A Sample Running Day Menu (for Me)

The menu below is actually what I've eaten before a 10-mile long run. The goal is to show you that you can eat for your sport while still being flexible. We are all doing our best with what we know and what we have in our fridge. Also, diet culture will have you believing that you can eat only boneless, skinless chicken breast and steamed green beans. Naw, let's get into it.

Dinner the Night Before

- Thai fried rice with shrimp
- Water

Pre-run Breakfast

- Two granola bars
- A banana

- Oatmeal
- Water
- Pre-workout supplements
  - Pre-workout powder free of caffeine and other stimulants
  - Vitamin B_{12}
  - Joint supplement (glucosamine and chondroitin)

On-the-Run Fuel

- 4 packets of energy chews
- Water/sports drink/hydration solution

Post-run Food

- Recovery protein shake
  - Two scoops of protein powder
  - One scoop of glutamine
  - Two scoops of frozen fruit
  - Water
- Two capsules of krill oil supplements
- Barbecued smoked sausage (My father-in-law was grilling when I was done running, so that's what I had!)
- Water/sports drink/hydration solution

2 Hours Post-run

- Ribs, macaroni and cheese, baked beans, asparagus, zucchini
- Water/sports drink/hydration solution

4 Hours Post-run

- Chicken shawarma with rice and salad
- Water/sports drink/hydration solution

As you can probably tell, the above menu is far from what diet culture might deem acceptable. I am calling some serious BS on that. The truth is, you gotta eat what's in your kitchen and what you have access to financially and geographically. As stated earlier, I take supplements under direct supervision of my nutritionist and healthcare provider, but that doesn't mean that you should start taking them. Consult your healthcare provider for YOUR best course of action.

The goal is to understand the basics so that you can incorporate your own version of running nutrition into your actual life. Got it? Don't be afraid of food or enjoying what you eat. It's one of the greatest tools you have when trying to become the best runner you can be.

RUNNING NUTRITION QUESTIONS ASKED BY EVERY BEGINNER, NONTRADITIONAL, SLOW, OR FAT RUNNER

1. **Why are carbohydrates so important?**

    Carbs are the building block of energy. They are the best energy source for our bodies while we are running.

2. **What is best to eat before a run?**

    Everyone's body is a bit different. The key is to have something high in carbs and protein but low in fat and fiber before a run. My personal favorite is a banana and peanut butter and jelly sandwich on whole wheat toast, or oatmeal.

3. **What are the best foods for recovery?**

    Again, everyone is different. Generally you want something that has carbs and protein within 30 to 60 minutes of working out. That is when your body is the most primed to take in nutrients.

Also, it helps prevent your body from leaching from your muscles to replace the nutrients that were depleted. As for recovery foods, I personally like to have a shake after my workout because I find that sometimes I am not hungry and a shake helps me get in the nutrients without eating. However, 2 hours after the workout I'm ready to throw down. So pasta is my go-to, and of course, carrot cake.

4. **Do I need to drink on the run?**

Unless you want to risk getting dehydrated, you should be drinking water or some type of sports drink on your run. Hydrate early and often. Never wait until you feel thirsty because generally that's too late.

5. **Do I need to carb-load, and if so, when should I start?**

When you're just starting out, no you don't need to carb-load. That's an advanced strategy for marathon runners. That's a topic for another book!

6. **Do runners require a special diet?**

Runners just need to pay attention to fueling their bodies properly, as I've outlined in this chapter. But of course everyone is a little different, and you may find you have different dietary requirements or needs. Maybe you'll thrive with more protein or more carbs in your diet, for example. Eat in a way that powers your runs effectively and suits your budget, lifestyle, and personal taste.

7. **Do I need to take any supplements?**

When you are starting out, no, you don't need any supplements. However, that should be a conversation between your healthcare provider and you. Now, if you're thinking you need to take supplements because it's going to make you a faster runner and make you ten years younger, then it's probably diet culture trying to sell you stuff. Just follow the guidelines in this chapter and you should be good to go.

8. How do I know if I should consider supplements?

Talk to a registered dietitian. Also, you can talk to your primary care physician and get blood work done to see if you are deficient in any nutrients.

9. Are my nutritional needs the same no matter if I'm a new or an experienced runner?

No, the distance and frequency you run will definitely have an effect on your nutritional needs. Also, other factors such as your speed, the intensity of the workout, and even the weather should be considered as well. For example, say you run 3 miles in 1 hour and 15 minutes and someone else ran that same distance in 30 minutes. Even though you both ran the same distance, you are running for a longer period of time, so you will need more calories and water than the other runner. The same can also be true for various weather conditions. Running in 70-degree weather with 87 percent humidity is not the same as running in 70-degree weather with 5 percent humidity in direct sunlight. Your body will perform differently under those two conditions, and you will have to tweak your nutrition to meet the needs of your body. This is why it's important to work with a nutritionist.

For more inspiration and examples on how to fuel your runs, check out chapter 4 of your Slow AF Run Club Bonus Companion Course, which you can get access to at slowafrunclub.com/course.

CHAPTER 5

Train the F*ck Up

Cautionary Tale: That Time I Almost Died

The year before the onset of the COVID-19 pandemic, I ran four marathons in a two-month span. This meant I had to train during the dog days of summer.

On one particular run, I was out for a 20-miler. I headed out around nine A.M., which was later than I should have left. I thought it was going to be a mild day. Instead, it turned out to be the hottest day of the year.

Initially I was killing it. I was running faster than my goal race pace and feeling good. At the end of the first 10 miles, I did the same thing I always do—went to the local fast-food joint. I used the restroom, refilled my water pack, had a snack, and headed out to run again. It was way hotter than before I had headed inside for a break. Still, I kept going. I was feeling great.

What I really loved about the trail I'd chosen that day was the abundance of shade, water fountains, and clean restrooms. I'd stop at every other fountain and check to make sure I had hydration and fuel and that I was still feeling good.

Around mile 15, I stopped to get water and fuel up. All I could think about was how hot it was outside. I wasn't worried, though— I was 5 miles from my car and feeling strong.

At this point the sun was high in the sky, going full blast. There was no shade in sight and the next water stop wasn't for another 2 miles. My pace slowed. I was drinking more water than I had during all the water stops.

Mile 17 finally came, and so did another fountain. I sat in the shade for a few minutes to cool down, drank some water, and had some more fuel.

As I sat there, I checked my hydration vest, and at that point it was half full. I didn't want to go through the hassle of filling it up and bogging myself down. I decided I'd do that at the next stop. Big mistake—I shouldn't have listened to myself.

I kept running. I'd been out there for hours. I still felt good, but my pace had slowed to a walk because it was 83 degrees Fahrenheit but felt like 95.

It felt like I was losing more water than I could take in. I was about half a mile from the next fountain when I heard the airy slurp of the hydration pack. No more water. No worries, though, right? The next station wasn't that far off! The sun was relentlessly beating down on me. I was starting to breathe heavily, and my mouth was drier than the Sahara.

I tried some positive self-talk. *Stay calm, Martinus, you're almost there, and you can get water and cool down for the last 2 miles.* The dryness moved into my throat. As much as I tried to stay calm, panic started to set in. I was starting to feel weak and light-headed.

That's when I saw this couple and, in a frantic state, told them that I was about to pass out and I needed water. The guy looked at me sideways. He told me to get out of there. He called me a bum.

I stopped another couple and told them what was happening.

"I'm training for a marathon. I've been out here for quite a bit and I ran out of water."

They gave me their water and suggested I sit under a tree and cool down. As I went to sit down, everything went black.

When I came to, I was surrounded by a group of people. Someone had taken off my shoes and socks. A park ranger asked me if I knew my name and what day it was. As I told him what had happened, he gave me water. I had some snacks in my bag, so I ate them until I felt better. Every time I tried to stand up, I felt dizzy. (I don't know why no one ever called an ambulance.) I sat under that dang tree until I felt better.

Eventually I was able to stand up without feeling dizzy, and the park ranger gave me a ride to my car. Then and there I knew something about my training was going to have to change. That day could have been the end of my life.

Remember, this happened in 2019. I'd been running for YEARS and still made these mistakes. I'm telling you now so that hopefully, you don't have to experience what I did.

Once you finally take the leap to train for a race, things in your running routine will be different. In this chapter I'm going to share some lessons that I learned from training during the past ten years and give you training plans to get you up and going. Let's go!

Training Logistics: Where to Run

The Great Outdoors

The training plans you'll find later in this chapter are meant to be used outdoors. Reason being that if you're planning on running a race in the future, nine times out of ten it's going to be outside on a road or trail. I'm not saying that you can't use these plans indoors, but for most runners, the action happens outside. That's a good thing!

Part of the pleasure of running outdoors is that it breaks up the monotony of running on a treadmill. You're out in the open air, under the sky, moving through the world. Even though you're more vulnerable to being heckled and other environmental hazards, it's worth it. Trust me.

While we are on the topic of heckling, let's talk about running outside in a larger body. It's not easy. It can be nerve-racking, but trust me. Do the thing.

Sometimes your mind will play tricks on you. Sometimes you are going to be hella self-conscious because you're out there doing the thing. You may have impostor syndrome. You may or may not find people looking at you. You may even get the occasional honk from a car. Sometimes assholes will shout and you might hear them. But you can get up and keep going. I say this with my whole chest:

Fuck. Them.

I'm telling you these things now so you can get mentally prepared.

For some of you reading this book, running outside will be downright scary or even seem impossible. Shake that off.

YOU GOT THIS. YOU BELONG HERE. No matter what happens, good or bad, I want you to know that running is for everyone. The outdoors are for all of us, people of every size, color, and age.

If you are still struggling with insecurity, there are a few things that you can do to help defend yourself from the outside world. For example, put on some headphones with your favorite tunes to get you hyped up and block people out. Running early in the morning when there aren't many people outside can help until you build up your confidence. Try the local track or a vacant parking lot. Remember, you have nothing to hide. Lastly, bring your "fuck the world" attitude. You are running for yourself, not for anyone else.

The Pavement, aka Streets and Sidewalks

Probably the most common place where runners run is on pavement. If you ever run a race, it'll most likely be on the road, so you might as well get used to it!

However, even if you limit yourself to pavement, the possibilities are endless. Going for a run is how I like to explore new places like vacation spots or my new neighborhood after a move.

Note, though, that it's true what they say: pavement is also the toughest on your body both physically and mentally. You'll also have to handle the elements—the heat, rain, sleet, snow, hail, smoke, and pollution. Sometimes you run into a stray dog, a possum, or a rat (shout-out to my New York City runners). Occasionally there are people to watch out for—keep your head on a swivel.

If you're heading to the pavement for the first time, be sure to find a flat stretch with less traffic that has plenty of shoulder space or a dedicated bike lane so you can step to the side to avoid oncoming traffic. Many runners I know got their start just by running to the corner of their block and back. Everyone starts somewhere.

> **Pro Tip:** Whether you're on the sidewalk or road, always run facing the traffic so you can see the cars coming. Make sure they can see you, too. For extra visibility, be sure to wear bright and/or reflective gear, especially before dawn and around or after dusk. I know some of you might be struggling with confidence, but trust me, you want to be seen. It's about safety.

The Outdoor Track

If you can find a track nearby, it would be an ideal place to start if you're new to running. Tracks are perfectly flat, and there's no concern about oncoming traffic. The distance is measured, and most tracks are softer than pavement.

However, tracks connected to schools usually have times when you can't use them, so you'll want to call ahead to get their schedule. The other thing about tracks? They can get boring, especially if you're spending anything longer than an hour going in circles, seeing the same thing over and over again.

As you progress in your running journey, the track is great for speed workouts, which you'll want to try to work into your routine when you can.[1] Often, a running club will meet at a track once a week (aka track Tuesday) to work on speed workouts.

Helpful Standard Track Measurements

- 100 meters: the length of the straightaway or curve
- 200 meters: the combined length of the straightaway and curve
- 400 meters: the length of 1 lap around the track
- 800 meters: about ½ mile or 2 laps around the track
- 1,600 meters: about 1 mile or 4 laps around the track

Trails

An unpaved trail (gravel or dirt) has a surface softer than pavement. It is a great place to run if you struggle with some injuries or joint irritation. However, you have to be cognizant of the trail's composition, because of roots, rocks, and uneven terrain. If you're an absolute beginner or are clumsy, skip unpaved trails for now because they could be more harmful than helpful.

The Great Indoors

As a runner, you have to be adaptable. Sometimes when you're training for a race, inclement weather can keep you from running outdoors. It can be dangerously hot or cold. You may have too much snow or ice,

---

[1] Note: If you're an absolute beginner, I would recommend you work on building your strength and distance first. If you add speed workouts before your body is ready, you could injure yourself.

or even too much smoke (shout-out to my California runners). Nature will try to hit you with everything it's got. Sometimes nature wins, and that's when running indoors comes into play.

You don't have to wait for better weather to run. To be honest, indoors isn't my favorite place to run, but it will do in a pinch.

Treadmill

The treadmill is a great starting point if you're an absolute beginner and you're not ready to start running outdoors. It provides a safe and convenient way to run.

Since the treadmill is a cushioned moving platform, you don't feel the pressures of gravity on your body. It is also clear of any obstacles like uneven terrain, rocks, oncoming traffic, and stray dogs. Make sure you run with at least a 1 to 2 percent incline on the treadmill; this setting will give you a feeling similar to running outside. Watch some TV or run to music, and your miles can fly by quickly.

> **Warning:** Sometimes the treadmill can turn into the dread-mill. It will make you feel like you're running on a hamster wheel if you run longer than 45 minutes to an hour on it. This is why it's kind of a last resort for many runners.

Lastly, most treadmills are not calibrated, so you may find your treadmill distances are off or don't match up to what you are running outside. In my experience, the treadmill is usually off by a quarter mile to half a mile. It may seem like you're running faster than you truly are, and MOST of the time the paces and distances are not equivalent to those outdoors. Don't get discouraged if this happens to you!

There are a few ways for you to deal with this. I find the best method to use when running on a treadmill is to focus on time rather than distance.

Most sports watches and running apps have a way to calibrate themselves to the treadmills that you are running on. This means you would have to run first and then input in the app what the distance says on the treadmill.

Indoor Track

You'll probably have one of these at your local YMCA, gym, or high school. If you don't mind running in circles for an hour inside, then this could be the option for you. These tracks have all the cushy benefits of the outdoor ones, but you usually need a paid membership of some kind to get access to them. Indoor tracks may also be smaller than outdoor ones. Smaller circles, more boredom.

Mapping Out Your Routes

This is something that I wish someone taught me when it came to running outside: how to map out a route.

I have a 1-mile route, 5K route, 5-mile route, and 10-mile route already mapped out around my neighborhood. I spent quite a bit of time planning them out so that when it's time to run I don't have to think about where I'm going. I know I have premeasured distances that are safe and have the amenities I need. I do run other places, but it's always good to have go-tos.

Finding Your Route

There are a couple of apps for that! Most fitness tracking apps like Strava, Garmin, Footpath, and MapMyRun usually have some type of heat map that shows the most popular places and routes that their users run.

You can also find places to run right under your nose. For example, is there a trail or path along the route that you go to work or the grocery store? Is there a local park you could run to, loop around, and head back home? Think about your neighborhood and its potential running paths and trails. You can also consult with your local run club and running shoe store about good running routes.

To be really thorough, check out your routes at different times during the day: early in the morning, at noon, in the evening. Over the course of a day, traffic can shift, and some areas may feel less safe closer to sundown. Ask yourself if you feel comfortable, and know the best times to run your routes.

Here are some other important factors to consider when picking your routes:

Is there any tree cover or shade? This is extremely important in the summer months (see the cautionary tale at the beginning of this chapter). Running in direct sunlight can suck the energy right out of you and be dangerous for your health. Sunburn. Heatstroke. Nah, thanks.

Will you have access to restrooms or Porta-Potties? Let me tell you something, you're gonna want to know where the public restrooms are at. Don't think it won't happen to you. One time I had to go number two in the bushes behind someone's house, and I used my sock as toilet paper. They saw me AND I finished the run with one sock. Not my proudest moment. #NeverPickUpARandomSock

Don't be like me; find all the places to do your bathroom business before you start running. You may want to run with toilet paper or wet wipes if said public restroom is sketchy on the toilet paper tip.

Will you have access to water? Is this route BYOW (Bring Your Own Water)? Are there places to refill or to buy an extra bottle if you need it? For shorter runs you may not need to worry about this, but in the summer and on longer outings, it's a MUST.

Is there a nearby road or extraction point? If you ever get hurt or need someone to pick you up, it's key to know how they will be able to get you. This is especially true if you are running on unpaved trails in the national parks.

Do you feel safe? Basically, does it feel safe to run in the area? Does it have lights and plenty of visibility? Is there a police presence? Are there stray dogs, coyotes, foxes, or rats roaming the streets? Are there people around who look like bad news? This is something that you'll have to personally gauge for yourself.

How close are you to home? Do you have to drive or take public transportation to get to the place where you're running? Take this into consideration when you are thinking about your longer runs. Do you want to start at your front door or do you want to travel, then run, and then travel back home?

Consider how much time that takes and your other obligations. As I said, I would definitely suggest having a route close to the home if possible for runs you want to take during the week.

Is there traffic? If you're running in urban areas such as New York City, you're going to encounter a lot of stoplights and traffic. This can make it tough to get in the groove while running. Are you okay with that? Or should you head to the park? Something to consider. Some people have no problem stopping and starting, while others need momentum. Figure out what works for you and plan your route accordingly.

Is it scenic? There's something about awe-inspiring views that help take your mind off running. Especially on those longer distances, green fields and blue skies can do the trick to make a 6-mile run feel less daunting.

Safety (When You Are Running Alone)

I want you to return home in the same shape that you left. I'm not trying to scare you, but safety is something that's easy to ignore until it happens to you, and by then it can be too late.

In my old neighborhood there was a string of attacks and robberies on the running trail I used to frequent. For the longest time I thought it couldn't happen to me because I'm a big guy. At least I thought that until one time I was on the trail with the volume of my music up too high and I didn't hear someone sneaking behind me. I didn't have anything on me but my phone, so I'm guessing that's why the person ended up running away. Still, I should have been vigilant so I wasn't relying on being lucky to keep me safe.

Sometimes these situations are not preventable, but you can do your best to protect yourself with the following tips.

1. **Be aware of your surroundings.** "Keep your head on a swivel" is a phrase that my high school football coach used to yell at us constantly. It means to be aware of your surroundings and constantly survey the scene at hand; you don't want to get blindsided by a player on the opposing team. This rings as true in running as it does in football.

   Keeping your head on a swivel means using all your senses to survey your surroundings. What do you see, hear, smell, and sense around you? This also means that you can't have your headphones blasting away. (Protect your hearing and stay safe!) I'm not saying that you can't wear headphones or earbuds, but try to keep the volume low. Or try running with only one earbud. You can also buy earbuds that have a transparency mode so you can hear what's happening around you. It's particularly important that you hear what's going on around you at dawn and dusk, when your visibility on a road or trail is more of an issue. Or go without the music! Some runners never run with headphones and prefer immersing themselves in their surroundings.

2. **Share your route with someone you trust.** Some apps will let you share your location with a friend or loved one. Just plug in the end point of your run and share the route with them (or several people). Taking this step could be the difference between life and death, and not just if you are attacked. You could get injured, have a health emergency, or have another kind of accident.

3. **Give them an estimate of how long the run should take.** An ETA gives your significant other, family member, or friend an idea of when you are going to be done with your run and back in contact. If they don't hear from you long after that projected ETA, that's a sign they should be worried. Don't forget to check back in with your person once your run is done in order to avoid freaking them out.

4. **Give periodic updates or calls.** When I'm running for longer than an hour and a half, I like to give updates on my run. Sometimes I'll do this on social media, or other times I'll call someone and share how I'm feeling, where I am, and how much longer I have to go. I like leaving bread crumbs just in case something happens.

Running at Dawn or Dusk

If you run early or late in the day, you want to be sure you are visible to others and protected at the same time. Here are a few items to carry:

- Headlamp
- Strobe lights
- Reflective gear
- Alarms/whistles
- Mace/pocketknife

- **Note:** You won't likely have to use these (I hope), but if it makes you feel safer to have them, then please carry them. Make sure you check your local laws about carrying Mace because it could be illegal to do so.

I said it before and I'll say it again: if you are running on the road, be sure to run against the flow of traffic.

Running While Black

Being a big Black man who is also a runner means I have more run-ins with the police than I want to. I've been cuffed, slammed on the hoods of police cruisers, and had guns drawn on me all because I "looked suspicious" or was outside during a time when I wasn't "supposed" to be.

The murder of twenty-five-year-old runner Ahmaud Arbery in 2020 damn near broke me. I almost hung up my running shoes for good because of it.

Running while Black can be a very sticky situation. Sometimes I have to get creative to make my six-three, 300-plus-pound Black body look less intimidating. I know making the people around me more comfortable could be the difference between life and death. That is why I sometimes run with my 10-pound poodle, Mabel, aka Clearance Puppy. I figure that people won't think someone who is threatening would be running with something so cute. (This is also the reason why the Slow AF Run Club turtle mascot is so cute. It's nonthreatening.) I also make a point to wear the brightest clothes I can find. I make sure what I'm doing can't be misconstrued.

There are times when I need to start running right before dusk. I wear all the safety equipment I listed above: headlamp, reflectors, strobe lights, and so forth. I run at various times of the day. I make it my business to introduce myself to my neighbors. People know me as "the big man who runs in the neighborhood." I always have my ID on me when I run. Always.

Though I wish I didn't feel the need to do these things, I understand it's for my own safety. It's all about giving myself the best opportunity to make it home in the same shape that I left. That's the reality of being a Black runner. To Black runners reading this book: These tips are some things to keep you safe. Don't be discouraged.

How to Be an Ally for Black Runners When Shit Is Hitting the Fan

- If you are white, use your whiteness as a shield of protection. What does this mean? Sometimes physically putting yourself in between the person being targeted and the aggressor is just enough to de-escalate the situation.
- Don't be the dick or the Karen to call the police on someone who is just living their life.
- Record the incident on your phone (but be careful).
- Vocally advocate for the person being targeted.

Other Running Tips: Things to Bring on a Run

Now we've talked about safety, let's get into what you actually need to bring on most runs. First of all, I always bring my cell phone, earbuds, ID or ROAD iD or something that has my name, my address, and my emergency contact info, and credit card or cash. Beyond that, I take what I'll need depending on how long I'll be out.

For 1 to 4 Miles, or up to 1 Hour of Running

For this distance you probably just need a water bottle. You may not even take a sip from it, but it's nice to have the option.

For 4 to 7 Miles, or 1 Hour up to 2 Hours of Running

For up to 2 hours of running I bring my water bottle, and I have a place in mind to refill the water bottle. You may want to bring a couple of fuel packs. I usually bring two, but I may not use both. See what works for you.

For 8 to 13 Miles, or 2 Hours up to 3 Hours of Running

For anything more than 2 hours of running, consider a hydration vest or backpack. I'll take at least a 1.5- to 2-liter bladder filled with just water or a sports drink/hydration mixture, also known as an electrolyte drink. Think Gatorade, Powerade, Skratch Labs, and Nuun Hydration. These drinks contain electrolytes, such as sodium, calcium, chloride, magnesium, phosphate, and potassium. These minerals help regulate the water in your body, so you can effectively get nutrients into your cells and waste out of your body. (If I fill the bladder with just water, I may bring a separate water bottle with a concentrated hydration solution in it.)

It can also be a good idea to carry the following:

- Imodium/Pepto Bismol chewables
- Baby wipes or body wipes
- Aspirin or some type of pain reliever
- Band-Aids
- Fuel packets
- Salt tablets (just in case you are losing more salt than you can replace)
- Anti-chafe lube

I call this my traveling pharmacy. These are the things that I used to stop and buy on a run during my more than ten years of running. Now I just have 'em on deck.

For 13 Miles or More, or 3 Hours of Running and Beyond

At this distance I bring my traveling pharmacy and a 3-liter bladder of water. I also pack a water bottle with a highly concentrated hydration solution. It's good to have a few places in mind where you can refill your hydration pack and water bottle.

OKAY. Either you've skipped up to this point or NOW you've learned all the safety tips and put together your gear! It's time to start running!

Your First Training Plan

Your First Week as a Runner

Welcome to the first week of your new running life! This week is about building consistency. You're not trying to work on speed, distances, or any of that fancy stuff you've read in any of the magazines.

Your goal when you're starting is to **get your ass outside and run at least three times this week**. You are building a new habit, and building new habits is hard. That's why your focus should be on getting out there.

You're excited! You're motivated, but you have to curb your enthusiasm and keep things measured. Many new runners do too much, too soon, then get injured. Nope! That's not going to be you. Diet culture and social media "rise and grind" BS has got you thinking that you need to jump into the deep end headfirst. Nah! Patience is key.

Give your body time to acclimatize to the new demands that you are putting on it. It takes a few weeks of *consistency* for your body to get used to something new.

If you're an absolute beginner and don't know where to start, here's what you need to know:

Your First Run

Warm up by walking for 5 minutes. Try running for **15 to 30 seconds** and then walking for **60 to 90 seconds**. Repeat until you can do this for at least **20 minutes** total. Do this three days a week for the first two weeks. Then start to increase the minutes to **30 minutes** for another two to three weeks and then try doing it for **45 minutes**.

After Your First Month

You're a month into the game now and the goal is still consistency. Keep at it. Around this point you can start to play around with the sliders of running to push yourself.

What Are the Sliders of Running?

These are things that you can adjust during your running workout:

- Run interval time/distance
- Run interval speed
- Walk interval time/distance
- Walk interval speed
- Total duration or distance of the run

When I'm coaching my clients, we work on adjusting these sliders so that they get the most out of their training and keep progressing. Here's an example. Say you've been doing 15-second running intervals alternating with 60-second walk intervals for a total duration of 30 minutes, three times a week for the past three weeks. On the fourth week, you can try increasing your run intervals to 30 or 45 seconds *or* you can decrease your walk intervals down to 45 or 30 seconds *or* you can increase the total duration of your run to 45 minutes to push yourself. You are probably thinking, *Martinus, which change should I make first?* Well, theoretically you can pick any one of those options to do first; just don't make more than one change at once. I know that answer won't be enough for everyone, so let's break it down. If you feel like the runs are too easy or hard or too short or long, then adjust the run interval time or distance or the run interval speed. If you feel like the walking breaks are too long and you recover faster or alternatively you need more time to recover, then adjust the walk interval time or distance or the walk interval speed. If you feel like the run and walk intervals are just right, then adjust the total duration or distance of the run. Making these small shifts will pay off in a big way and get you where you need to go.

After Your First Three Months

Okay, you're three months in the game. Look at you go! At this point, you're a running machine, and you probably are craving a challenge or goal. It's time to consider training for or running a 5K. For that, you'll need a training plan. Your boy Martinus got you covered. See below to get started! If you feel like you need more time before training for a 5K, you'll find a four-week base-building training plan to get you started. If you feel like you have already mastered the 5K distance, you'll find a 10K training plan below. Pick out the plan that best fits your fitness level and goals. Be realistic.

Four-Week Base-Building Training Plan

This is a precursor to the 5K training plan. If you feel like you've been out of the game too long, this plan will help prime you for 5K training.

	Day 1	Day 2	Day 3	Day 4	Day 5	Day 6	Day 7
Week 1	Warm up 5–10 minutes. Run: 15 seconds. Walk: 90 seconds. Repeat 10 times. Cooldown.	Rest Day and/or Stretching Day	Warm up 5–10 minutes. Run: 15 seconds. Walk: 90 seconds. Repeat 10 times. Cooldown.	Rest Day and/or Cross-Training Day	Rest Day and/or Stretching Day	Warm up 5–10 minutes. Run: 15 seconds. Walk: 90 seconds. Repeat 15 times. Cooldown.	Rest Day and/or Cross-Training Day
Week 2	Warm up 5–10 minutes. Run: 15 seconds. Walk: 90 seconds. Repeat 15 times. Cooldown.	Rest Day and/or Stretching Day	Warm up 5–10 minutes. Run: 15 seconds. Walk: 90 seconds. Repeat 20 times. Cooldown.	Rest Day and/or Cross-Training Day	Rest Day and/or Stretching Day	Warm up 5–10 minutes. Run: 15 seconds. Walk: 90 seconds. Repeat 20 times. Cooldown.	Rest Day and/or Cross-Training Day

	Day 1	Day 2	Day 3	Day 4	Day 5	Day 6	Day 7
Week 3	Warm up 5–10 minutes. Run: 30 seconds. Walk: 90 seconds. Repeat 15 times. Cooldown.	Rest Day and/or Stretching Day	Warm up 5–10 minutes. Run: 30 seconds. Walk: 90 seconds. Repeat 15 times. Cooldown.	Rest Day and/or Cross-Training Day	Rest Day and/or Stretching Day	Warm up 5–10 minutes. Run: 30 seconds. Walk: 90 seconds. Repeat 20 times. Cooldown.	Rest Day and/or Cross-Training Day
Week 4	Warm up 5–10 minutes. Run: 30 seconds. Walk: 90 seconds. Repeat 20 times. Cooldown.	Rest Day and/or Stretching Day	Warm up 5–10 minutes. Run: 45 seconds. Walk: 90 seconds. Repeat 15 times. Cooldown.	Rest Day and/or Cross-Training Day	Rest Day and/or Stretching Day	Warm up 5–10 minutes. Run: 45 seconds. Walk: 90 seconds. Repeat 15 times. Cooldown.	Rest Day and/or Cross-Training Day

Twelve-Week 5K Training Plan

	Day 1	Day 2	Day 3	Day 4	Day 5	Day 6	Day 7
Week 1	Warm up 5–10 minutes. Run: 1 minute. Walk: 2 minutes. Repeat 10 times. Cooldown.	Rest Day and/or Stretching Day	Warm up 5–10 minutes. Run: 1 minute. Walk: 2 minutes. Repeat 10 times. Cooldown.	Rest Day and/or Cross-Training Day	Rest Day and/or Stretching Day	Warm up 5–10 minutes. Run: 1 minute. Walk: 2 minutes. Repeat 10 times. Cooldown.	Rest Day and/or Cross-Training Day
Week 2	Warm up 5–10 minutes. Run: 1 minute. Walk: 2 minutes. Repeat 15 times. Cooldown.	Rest Day and/or Stretching Day	Warm up 5–10 minutes. Run: 1 minute. Walk: 2 minutes. Repeat 15 times. Cooldown.	Rest Day and/or Cross-Training Day	Rest Day and/or Stretching Day	Warm up 5–10 minutes. Run: 1.5 minutes. Walk: 2 minutes. Repeat 10 times. Cooldown.	Rest Day and/or Cross-Training Day

	Day 1	Day 2	Day 3	Day 4	Day 5	Day 6	Day 7
Week 3	Warm up 5–10 minutes. Run: 1.5 minutes. Walk: 2 minutes. Repeat 10 times. Cooldown.	Rest Day and/or Stretching Day	Warm up 5–10 minutes. Run: 1.5 minutes. Walk: 1.5 minutes. Repeat 15 times. Cooldown.	Rest Day and/or Cross-Training Day	Rest Day and/or Stretching Day	Warm up 5–10 minutes. Run: 1.5 minutes. Walk: 1.5 minutes. Repeat 15 times. Cooldown.	Rest Day and/or Cross-Training Day
Week 4	Warm up 5–10 minutes. Run: 2 minutes. Walk: 2 minutes. Repeat 8 times. Cooldown.	Rest Day and/or Stretching Day	Warm up 5–10 minutes. Run: 2 minutes. Walk: 2 minutes. Repeat 8 times. Cooldown.	Rest Day and/or Cross-Training Day	Rest Day and/or Stretching Day	Warm up 5–10 minutes. Run: 2 minutes. Walk: 2 minutes. Repeat 10 times. Cooldown.	Rest Day and/or Cross-Training Day
Week 5	Warm up 5–10 minutes. Run: 2 minutes. Walk: 2 minutes. Repeat 10 times. Cooldown.	Rest Day and/or Stretching Day	Warm up 5–10 minutes. Run: 2 minutes. Walk: 1.5 minutes. Repeat 13 times. Cooldown.	Rest Day and/or Cross-Training Day	Rest Day and/or Stretching Day	Warm up 5–10 minutes. Run: 2 minutes. Walk: 1.5 minutes. Repeat 13 times. Cooldown.	Rest Day and/or Cross-Training Day
Week 6	Warm up 5–10 minutes. Run: 2 minutes. Walk: 1.5 minutes. Repeat 15 times. Cooldown.	Rest Day and/or Stretching Day	Warm up 5–10 minutes. Run: 2 minutes. Walk: 1 minute. Repeat 15 times. Cooldown.	Rest Day and/or Cross-Training Day	Rest Day and/or Stretching Day	Warm up 5–10 minutes. Run: 2 minutes. Walk: 1 minute. Repeat 15 times. Cooldown.	Rest Day and/or Cross-Training Day

	Day 1	Day 2	Day 3	Day 4	Day 5	Day 6	Day 7
Week 7	Warm up 5–10 minutes. Run: 3 minutes. Walk: 2 minutes. Repeat 6 times. Cooldown.	Rest Day and/or Stretching Day	Warm up 5–10 minutes. Run: 3 minutes. Walk: 2 minutes. Repeat 6 times. Cooldown.	Rest Day and/or Cross-Training Day	Rest Day and/or Stretching Day	Warm up 5–10 minutes. Run: 3 minutes. Walk: 2 minutes. Repeat 8 times. Cooldown.	Rest Day and/or Cross-Training Day
Week 8	Warm up 5–10 minutes. Run: 3 minutes. Walk: 2 minutes. Repeat 8 times. Cooldown.	Rest Day and/or Stretching Day	Warm up 5–10 minutes. Run: 3 minutes. Walk: 1.5 minutes. Repeat 10 times. Cooldown.	Rest Day and/or Cross-Training Day	Rest Day and/or Stretching Day	Warm up 5–10 minutes. Run: 3 minutes. Walk: 1.5 minutes. Repeat 10 times. Cooldown.	Rest Day and/or Cross-Training Day
Week 9	Warm up 5–10 minutes. Run: 3 minutes. Walk: 1.5 minutes. Repeat 10 times. Cooldown.	Rest Day and/or Stretching Day	Warm up 5–10 minutes. Run: 3 minutes. Walk: 1 minute. Repeat 12 times. Cooldown.	Rest Day and/or Cross-Training Day	Rest Day and/or Stretching Day	Warm up 5–10 minutes. Run: 3 minutes. Walk: 1 minute. Repeat 12 times. Cooldown.	Rest Day and/or Cross-Training Day
Week 10	Warm up 5–10 minutes. Run: 4 minutes. Walk: 2 minutes. Repeat 6 times. Cooldown.	Rest Day and/or Stretching Day	Warm up 5–10 minutes. Run: 4 minutes. Walk: 2 minutes. Repeat 6 times. Cooldown.	Rest Day and/or Cross-Training Day	Rest Day and/or Stretching Day	Warm up 5–10 minutes. Run: 4 minutes. Walk: 2 minutes. Repeat 8 times. Cooldown.	Rest Day and/or Cross-Training Day

	Day 1	Day 2	Day 3	Day 4	Day 5	Day 6	Day 7
Week 11	Warm up 5–10 minutes. Run: 4 minutes. Walk: 2 minutes. Repeat 8 times. Cooldown.	Rest Day and/or Stretch-ing Day	Warm up 5–10 minutes. Run: 4 minutes. Walk: 2 minutes. Repeat 10 times. Cooldown.	Rest Day and/or Cross-Training Day	Rest Day and/or Stretch-ing Day	Warm up 5–10 minutes. Run: 4 minutes. Walk: 1.5 minutes. Repeat 10 times. Cooldown.	Rest Day and/or Cross-Training Day
Week 12	Warm up 5–10 minutes. Run: 4 minutes. Walk: 1.5 minutes. Repeat 10 times. Cooldown.	Rest Day and/or Stretch-ing Day	Warm up 5–10 minutes. Run: 4 minutes. Walk: 1 minute. Repeat 10 times. Cooldown.	Rest Day and/or Cross-Training Day	Rest Day and/or Stretch-ing Day	Warm up 5–10 minutes. Run: 4 minutes. Walk: 1 minute. Repeat until 5K. Cooldown.	Rest Day and/or Cross-Training Day

Twelve-Week 10K Training Plan

	Day 1	Day 2	Day 3	Day 4	Day 5	Day 6	Day 7
Week 1	Warm up 5–10 minutes. Run: 1 minute. Walk: 2 minutes. Repeat 17 times. Cooldown.	Rest Day and/or Stretch-ing Day	Warm up 5–10 minutes. Run: 1 minute. Walk: 2 minutes. Repeat 17 times. Cooldown.	Rest Day and/or Cross-Training Day	Warm up 5–10 minutes. Run: 1.5 minutes. Walk: 2 minutes. Repeat 17 times. Cooldown.	Rest Day and/or Stretch-ing Day	Warm up 5–10 minutes. Run: 1.5 minutes. Walk: 2 minutes. Repeat 17 times. Cooldown.
Week 2	Warm up 5–10 minutes. Run: 2 minutes. Walk: 2 minutes. Repeat 12 times. Cooldown.	Rest Day and/or Stretch-ing Day	Warm up 5–10 minutes. Run: 2 minutes. Walk: 2 minutes. Repeat 12 times. Cooldown.	Rest Day and/or Cross-Training Day	Warm up 5–10 minutes. Run: 2 minutes. Walk: 2 minutes. Repeat 15 times. Cooldown.	Rest Day and/or Stretch-ing Day	Warm up 5–10 minutes. Run: 2 minutes. Walk: 2 minutes. Repeat 15 times. Cooldown.

	Day 1	Day 2	Day 3	Day 4	Day 5	Day 6	Day 7
Week 3	Warm up 5–10 minutes. Run: 2.5 minutes. Walk: 2.5 minutes. Repeat 9 times. Cooldown.	Rest Day and/or Stretching Day	Warm up 5–10 minutes. Run: 2.5 minutes. Walk: 2.5 minutes. Repeat 9 times. Cooldown.	Rest Day and/or Cross-Training Day	Warm up 5–10 minutes. Run: 2.5 minutes. Walk: 2.5 minutes. Repeat 9 times. Cooldown.	Rest Day and/or Stretching Day	Warm up 5–10 minutes. Run: 2.5 minutes. Walk: 2.5 minutes. Repeat 11 times. Cooldown.
Week 4	Warm up 5–10 minutes. Run: 2.5 minutes. Walk: 2.5 minutes. Repeat 9 times. Cooldown.	Rest Day and/or Stretching Day	Warm up 5–10 minutes. Run: 3 minutes. Walk: 2 minutes. Repeat 10 times. Cooldown.	Rest Day and/or Cross-Training Day	Warm up 5–10 minutes. Run: 3 minutes. Walk: 2 minutes. Repeat 10 times. Cooldown.	Rest Day and/or Stretching Day	Warm up 5–10 minutes. Run: 2.5 minutes. Walk: 2.5 minutes. Repeat 12 times. Cooldown.
Week 5	Warm up 5–10 minutes. Run: 3 minutes. Walk: 2 minutes. Repeat 9 times. Cooldown.	Rest Day and/or Stretching Day	Warm up 5–10 minutes. Run: 3 minutes. Walk: 2 minutes. Repeat 10 times. Cooldown.	Rest Day and/or Cross-Training Day	Warm up 5–10 minutes. Run: 3 minutes. Walk: 2 minutes. Repeat 10 times. Cooldown.	Rest Day and/or Stretching Day	Warm up 5–10 minutes. Run: 3 minutes. Walk: 2 minutes. Repeat 13 times. Cooldown.
Week 6	Warm up 5–10 minutes. Run: 3 minutes. Walk: 2 minutes. Repeat 10 times. Cooldown.	Rest Day and/or Stretching Day	Warm up 5–10 minutes. Run: 4 minutes. Walk: 2 minutes. Repeat 8 times. Cooldown.	Rest Day and/or Cross Training Day	Warm up 5–10 minutes. Run: 3 minutes. Walk: 2 minutes. Repeat 10 times. Cooldown.	Rest Day and/or Stretching Day	Warm up 5–10 minutes. Run: 3 minutes. Walk: 2 minutes. Repeat 14 times. Cooldown.

	Day 1	Day 2	Day 3	Day 4	Day 5	Day 6	Day 7
Week 7	Warm up 5–10 minutes. Run: 4 minutes. Walk: 2 minutes. Repeat 8 times. Cooldown.	Rest Day and/or Stretching Day	Warm up 5–10 minutes. Run: 4 minutes. Walk: 2 minutes. Repeat 10 times. Cooldown.	Rest Day and/or Cross-Training Day	Warm up 5–10 minutes. Run: 4 minutes. Walk: 2 minutes. Repeat 8 times. Cooldown.	Rest Day and/or Stretching Day	Warm up 5–10 minutes. Run: 4 minutes. Walk: 2 minutes. Repeat 13 times. Cooldown.
Week 8	Warm up 5–10 minutes. Run: 4 minutes. Walk: 2 minutes. Repeat 10 times. Cooldown.	Rest Day and/or Stretching Day	Warm up 5–10 minutes. Run: 4 minutes. Walk: 2 minutes. Repeat 10 times. Cooldown.	Rest Day and/or Cross-Training Day	Warm up 5–10 minutes. Run: 5 minutes. Walk: 2 minutes. Repeat 10 times. Cooldown.	Rest Day and/or Stretching Day	Warm up 5–10 minutes. Run: 4 minutes. Walk: 2 minutes. Repeat 14 times. Cooldown.
Week 9	Warm up 5–10 minutes. Run: 5 minutes. Walk: 2 minutes. Repeat 9 times. Cooldown.	Rest Day and/or Stretching Day	Warm up 5–10 minutes. Run: 5 minutes. Walk: 2 minutes. Repeat 11 times. Cooldown.	Rest Day and/or Cross-Training Day	Warm up 5–10 minutes. Run: 5 minutes. Walk: 2 minutes. Repeat 7 times. Cooldown.	Rest Day and/or Stretching Day	Warm up 5–10 minutes. Run: 5 minutes. Walk: 2 minutes. Repeat 13 times. Cooldown.
Week 10	Warm up 5–10 minutes. Run: 5 minutes. Walk: 2 minutes. Repeat 7 times. Cooldown.	Rest Day and/or Stretching Day	Warm up 5–10 minutes. Run: 5 minutes. Walk: 2 minutes. Repeat 12 times. Cooldown.	Rest Day and/or Cross-Training Day	Warm up 5–10 minutes. Run: 5 minutes. Walk: 2 minutes. Repeat 13 times. Cooldown.	Rest Day and/or Stretching Day	Warm up 5–10 minutes. Run: 4 minutes. Walk: 2 minutes. Repeat 15 times. Cooldown.

	Day 1	Day 2	Day 3	Day 4	Day 5	Day 6	Day 7
Week 11	Warm up 5–10 minutes. Run: 5 minutes. Walk: 2 minutes. Repeat 12 times. Cooldown.	Rest Day and/or Stretching Day	Warm up 5–10 minutes. Run: 5 minutes. Walk: 2 minutes. Repeat 15 times. Cooldown.	Rest Day and/or Cross-Training Day	Warm up 5–10 minutes. Run: 5 minutes. Walk: 2 minutes. Repeat 13 times. Cooldown.	Rest Day and/or Stretching Day	Warm up 5–10 minutes. Run: 5 minutes. Walk: 2 minutes. Repeat 17 times. Cooldown.
Week 12	Warm up 5–10 minutes. Run: 5 minutes. Walk: 1 minute. Repeat 12 times. Cooldown.	Rest Day and/or Stretching Day	Warm up 5–10 minutes. Run: 5 minutes. Walk: 1 minute. Repeat 16 times. Cooldown.	Rest Day and/or Cross-Training Day	Warm up 5–10 minutes. Run: 5 minutes. Walk: 1 minute. Repeat 13 times. Cooldown.	Rest Day and/or Stretching Day	Warm up 5–10 minutes. Run: 5 minutes. Walk: 1 minute. Repeat until 10K distance. Cooldown.

Missing Workouts/Runs

I'll keep this one brief. Rule of thumb: Never miss two workouts in a row. The first time is just life, but the second one is the start of a new habit. Now, if you're sick or injured, that's another thing.[2] Do what you need to do to get well first.

Warm-Up and Cooldown

The Warm-Up

Warming up both your body and mind are crucial to staying healthy and building up a strong base as a runner.

---

[2] If you're injured and your body allows it, you still should cross-train other body parts. There's still a benefit to doing that. (See chapter 8 for more.)

Warming Up the Mind

One of the things I recommend is developing a mental warm-up routine. I have a mindfulness practice that I do before each run, which involves rehearsing for the real thing in my head. If it's a race, I visualize the finish line. If it's a long run or a jog around the block, I imagine smooth, seamless motion.

Before You Run

- Scan your body from head to toe.
  - Note any areas that might need attention. Is anything tight or achy? Does it need extra stretching?
  - Note how you're feeling mentally. Are you in the zone and ready to go? Do you need a mindset shift?

Warming Up the Body

Getting into the habit of warming up with dynamic stretching before a run and static stretching after your run is part of developing GOOD. RUNNING. HYGIENE! These are important practices to help you get stronger and prevent injury.

DYNAMIC STRETCHING VS. STATIC STRETCHING

There are two types of stretching runners can do, and each has its own unique purpose.

Dynamic Stretching: This consists of movement-based stretches that are important to do before a run. You want to wake up your muscles and joints for all the action ahead!

Static Stretching: This is what people often imagine when they think of stretching. It involves holding a pose or stretching for

60 to 90 seconds. It's best to perform static stretches when
your muscles are warm, and so you should do these stretches
after your run is complete.

There is no perfect way to warm up. There's even conflicting research on whether warming up is good for you. What I'll say is this: do
what feels right to you.

You can do a Google search for the perfect running warm-up routine, and you'll find that all the suggested routines will be different.
There is no right way or wrong way to warm up. These are just possible
different ways of doing it. Below I'm going to share with you my current warm-up routine. Start here and let your warm-up evolve when
you feel comfortable.

Note: If you're an absolute beginner, the workout may initially seem intimidating. If that's the case, start out with something as simple as
walking for 5 minutes before you launch into running. As you start to
feel more confident, you can eventually move into the warm-up below
to get your body ready for running.

Martinus's Warm-Up Routine

**Complete the first exercise and then move on to the second,
the third, and so forth until you're done with the circuit.**
Then repeat the circuit once you've finished all the sets that
you wanted to do. If you are looking for pictures and videos
about how to do these exercises, check out chapter 5 of the
Slow AF Run Club Bonus Companion Course at slowafrunclub
.com/course.

Perform two sets of 5 to 10 reps each.

Pre-run Stretches

1. Lateral lunges
2. Kang squats
3. Standing quad stretch
4. Hacky sack
5. Toe swipes
6. High knees
7. Butt kicks
8. Leg swings
9. Quick feet

For some of these exercises, I ask you to take an athletic stance. Here's what that looks like: Stand with your feet shoulder-width apart, your hips and knees slightly bent. Look straight ahead and keep your chest open. Lock your body into position by engaging your core, which involves drawing your belly button into your spine. (I always imagine that someone is about to punch me in the gut!) Then you're ready to roll.

1. **Lateral lunges.** Start by standing in your athletic stance. On an inhale, take a slow step to the left side. Keep your toes pointed forward. Allow your knee and hips to bend, moving your weight down and to the left in a side lunge. Pause for 1 to 3 seconds, and then on the exhale, straighten the bent leg to return to a standing position, transitioning into a lunge on the opposite side.

2. **Kang squats.** Start by standing in your athletic stance. Your hands should be either behind your head or crossed over your chest. Keeping your back flat, hinge at the hips and push your butt straight back. Lower your torso toward the floor until you notice a stretch in your hamstrings. Leading with your hips and butt, sit back as far as you can go. As you squat, keep your head and chest up and push your knees out. Then push

your heel through the ground until you return to the starting position.

3. **Standing quad stretch.** Start by standing in your athletic stance. Shift your weight to stand on your right foot and grab your left shin or ankle by bending your leg behind you. Tuck your pelvis in and pull your shin toward your glutes, making sure your knee is pointed toward the ground. Try not to pull the knee backward or sideways. If you feel unsteady, hold on to something for balance. Pause for a second. Then switch sides and repeat the exercise.

4. **Hacky sack.** Start by standing in your athletic stance. Lift your right knee up, bending it so it points out. Bring your foot in (as if you're kicking a hacky sack) and, without bending forward, use your left hand to tap the inside of your ankle. Alternate legs, keeping your core engaged throughout.

5. **Toe swipes.** Start by standing with your feet together. Take a step forward with your right foot, planting your heel on the ground and keeping your legs straight. With a flat back, hinge at the hips and push your butt straight back. Lower your torso toward the floor, swinging your arm from the back of your foot then forward and up, until you're standing straight. Then step forward with your left foot and repeat the exercise.

6. **High knees.** Start by standing in your athletic stance. Lift your right knee to your chest, grab your shin with your hands, and pull your leg up and toward your chest. Hold for a second. Release and repeat on the other side.

7. **Butt kicks.** Start by standing in your athletic stance. As you swing your left arm forward, tighten your hamstring and slowly kick your right heel up toward your right butt cheek. Place your right foot back on the floor and repeat with your left foot.

8. **Leg swings.** Extend your right arm out to your side to support yourself by holding on to a wall or anything else stable. Swing

your right leg forward and back, keeping it as straight as pos-sible. Engage your core and keep your trunk vertical as you move. Do the required reps with the right leg. Then turn around and do the same number of reps with the left.

9. **Quick feet.** Start by standing in your athletic stance. Staying on the balls of your feet, run in place quickly.

As you get more into running, you'll find all types of quirks in your body that need adjusting. For me, the warm-up is useful to tend to those quirks before I start running. You have tight calves? Maybe you want to do a few stretches to loosen them up. Tight shoulders? Roll 'em. Tight hamstrings? Get after them. You do you. The most important thing is to make it your own. It's an integral part of your running routine.

The Cooldown

Cooling down is important because it returns the body to a resting state. Cooldown exercises (such as stretches) can aid the process of releasing and removing lactic acid from your muscles, helping to speed up your body's recovery post-workout.

Plus this is a part of the journey of being an athlete. It's time to ENJOY, feel the endorphins, stand confident in your body, and cele-brate what you accomplished!

Don't miss out!

Martinus's Cooldown Routine

Turn off Garmin or any tracking device. Seriously, don't forget. You'll thank me later.

Easy jog or walk for 5 to 10 minutes or until you've caught your breath. Don't stop immediately after a hard workout or you'll risk cramping or dizziness. The key is to lower the heart rate gradually.

Hydrate and refuel. Sip some water and have a snack! This will replenish your fluids and help repair muscle damage. Try to snack within 20 to 30 minutes after your workout or race.

Stretch. Now is the time to do some static stretching to lengthen tight muscles and release the tension built up while running.

Post-run Stretches

1. Standing calf stretch
2. Standing quad stretch
3. Tensor fasciae latae (TFL) stretch
4. Forward fold
5. Cross-arm stretch
6. Overhead triceps stretch
7. Runner's lunge
8. Butterfly stretch

1. **Standing calf stretch.** Stand facing a wall. Extend your arms out in front of you, placing your hands on the wall. Keeping your back straight, step forward with your right foot and bend your knee, while leaving your left leg extended straight back. Be sure that both feet are flat on the floor, with your heels planted on the ground. Lean toward the wall to stretch the calf muscle in your left leg. Hold for the desired length of stretch. Switch legs and repeat.

2. **Standing quad stretch.** Start by standing in your athletic stance. Shift your weight to stand on your right foot and grab your left shin or ankle by bending your leg behind you. Tuck your pelvis in and pull your shin toward your butt, making sure your knee is pointing toward the ground. Try not to pull the knee backward or sideways. If you feel unsteady, hold

on to something for balance. Hold for the desired length of time. Then switch sides and repeat the exercise.

3. **Tensor fasciae latae (TFL) stretch.** Stand with your feet hip-width apart. Cross your right leg behind your left and place your right foot slightly behind and to the outside of your left heel. Lean to the left and reach your right arm overhead. You should feel a stretch in your right hip flexors and the side of your right hip and arm. Hold for the desired length of time. Switch legs and repeat.

4. **Forward fold.** Start by standing in your athletic stance. Keeping your back flat, fold forward, hinging at the hips and pushing your butt straight back. Lower your torso toward the floor while trying to touch the ground until you notice a stretch in your hamstrings. Hold for the desired length of time and repeat.

5. **Cross-arm stretch.** Keeping your shoulder down, bring your left arm across the chest. Hold your left elbow (or forearm or wrist) with your right hand and gently pull your left arm toward your body. Hold this stretch for the desired length of time. Switch arms and repeat.

6. **Overhead triceps stretch.** Extend your right arm straight toward the ceiling. Bend the arm at the elbow to bring your right palm toward the center of your back, resting your middle finger along your spine. Use your left hand to gently pull your elbow (or push against your triceps for leverage) in toward the center and down. Hold this stretch for the desired length of time and repeat on the other side.

7. **Runner's lunge.** Kneel on your left knee and place your right foot on the floor in front of you so the bend in your knee makes a 90-degree angle. Lean forward until you feel a stretch in the front of your left hip. You can use your arms to help you maintain your balance or place both hands on your right knee. Hold

this stretch for the desired length of time, then switch sides. (You can rest your hand on a chair or a low prop to perform this exercise.)

8. **Butterfly stretch.** Sit on the floor or ground with the soles of your feet pressed together. Grasp your feet with your hands and rest your elbows on your knees. While keeping your back straight (no slouching), allow your knees to fall toward the ground. You can apply gentle pressure on the inner thigh by pressing gently on the knees with the elbows. You should feel this stretch throughout your inner thighs, the outermost part of your hips, and your lower back. Hold this stretch for the desired length of time. Release and repeat three times.

Tracking Your Training

I mentioned this in chapter 2, and I'll give you another friendly reminder now: track your training. It's a great way to follow your own progress along the way. (It's also a great way to know how many miles you have run in your shoes, so you'll know when to replace them.) You don't know where you are going unless you know where you've been. While you are on your journey, here are a few things that you could track in a running journal:

- Time of day
- Duration
- Distance/mileage
- Pace
- What interval (if any)
- Weather
  - Temperature
  - Humidity
  - Precipitation

- How you are feeling mentally and physically
- Aches or pains
- Any other comments or concerns

Whatever form your running journal takes—a Google Doc, a note in your phone, an app, or an old-school paper record—it can be beneficial and fun for your running.

TRAINING QUESTIONS ASKED BY EVERY BEGINNER, NONTRADITIONAL, SLOW, OR FAT RUNNER

---

1. **Should I train for speed or distance first?**

It depends where you are on your journey. If you are very new to the game, I would say that it's most important to work on distance and consistency first. Doing speed work when your body is not acclimated is a first-class trip to Injuryville.

2. **When should I train for speed?**

I wouldn't add speed work to your training if you are an absolute beginner. Just run more and your body will get more efficient; then you will start to run faster naturally. I usually wait until after my clients have been training for eight to ten weeks before I add speed training to their workouts. That way they have time to get acclimated to running first. Then I incorporate pickups—running for a sustained period at a faster pace than they'd typically do—into their runs. So what does this look like? Say you're running a 2/1 interval, where you are running for 2 minutes and walking for 1 minute. I would have you run your first 30 seconds at your regular pace. Then I would ask you to run the next minute at a faster pace. Your last 30 seconds would be back to your regular pace.

3. **What if I just started but I feel like I should be doing more?**

That's perfectly normal. Trust the process. When you do too much, too soon, you get injured.

4. **What happens if I miss a week or month?**

It's okay to miss a day or a week and get back on track. Conventional wisdom says that it depends on the situation. If it's a shorter distance during the week, then it's probably okay to miss it. But if it's a long run, you probably don't want to miss it. I would probably suggest repeating that week in your training plan.

5. **Is there flexibility in the training plans? Do I have to follow the training plan to a tee?**

When it comes to training plans, not everything can be set in stone. Life is not perfect, so I don't expect your training cycle to be perfect. I'm certainly not perfect! I've been training for the Boston Marathon as I've been writing this book. I've missed workouts. Sometimes I've missed more than two in a row. One weekend I had two weddings and a birthday party to go to and I was scheduled to run 20 miles. Well, that weekend was shot, but I did the best I could. I ended up splitting the 20 miles into two days. Things like this are going to happen. **It's about being consistent, not being perfect.**

CHAPTER 6

Boss Up and Get That Race Medal

Cautionary (Inspirational) Tale: My First 5K

As soon as the alarm buzzed, I reached over to turn it off. I'd been awake for at least an hour, anxiously staring at the ceiling. It was RACE DAY—the day of my very first 5K. As I got up and dressed, Char, my significant other, asked how I was feeling. Playing it cool, I shrugged. Deep down inside, I was nervous as hell. I didn't know what to expect. I didn't know if the other runners would accept me. What would happen if I was the last person to finish the race? What if I got lost? What if they ran out of water? So many questions swirled in my head. *Get ahold of yourself, dude. You've done the training, and for god's sake, you already ran 3 miles the day before yesterday to see if you could do it and you pulled it off. There's nothing to worry about.* I said this to myself in the mirror as I brushed my teeth over and over.

When I got to Watrous Park in Connecticut, where the race was being held, there were hundreds of people there, ready to run. As I waited to be directed to the starting line, I noticed that I stood out like a sore thumb. A fat Black man wearing a bright orange shirt and shoes to match was getting ready to run a race in a sea of fit white people. I felt like all eyes were on me. I wasn't imagining it, either. It seemed like everyone wanted to talk to me.

"Those are some very bright shoes," a guy said to me.

"Thank you," I responded.

"Is this your first race?"

"Yes."

"Well, good luck." I smiled and nodded, nervously walking back to where I had parked my car, away from everyone else. I did my warm-up there, away from the eyes and questions. I felt out of place and out of my league. My thoughts were racing and I was full of nervous energy.

Making my way to the starting line, I went all the way to the back. I'm talking WAY back, passing everyone—the fast people in the front, the people in the middle of the pack, and even the people who were walking the race. I lined up behind the parents with strollers, including the ones with dogs attached to them. I was literally the very last person. I really thought I was the slowest runner out there. I really thought that a mom pushing a dual stroller with a dog attached to her hip would finish the race before me. (I'm not saying anything about the running ability of these women; they just had a lot going on. This shows how little confidence I really had in myself at the time.) I had done the training, I had run 3 miles two days before, and I still positioned myself as the last person in the race.

When the gun went off, I walked slowly behind the crowd of runners, patiently waiting to cross the starting line. When I finally did, I took off like a bat out of hell.

I spent the first 10 or so minutes dodging and passing the people with strollers who I had initially thought were faster than me. Then I passed the walkers. Then something odd happened: I started to pass other runners. *Holy shit, I'm really doing this running thing*, I thought, grinning from ear to ear. Around the first mile marker, I got in the zone and felt unstoppable. When I got to the halfway mark, I was getting high fives from the faster runners doubling back on their way to the finish line. During my last half mile, so close to the finish line, I kicked my pace into an even higher gear. That's when I started to pass a lot of people. At first it felt weird that I was running fast enough to pass anyone, but as I passed the fifth person, it felt great.

As I approached the finish line, everyone was cheering and clapping; all I could do was smile because I had done it. I had run a 5K! It was one of the greatest feelings I had experienced in a long time. I was extremely proud of myself. I came from falling off a treadmill on my first run to finishing my first 5K.

This is what it's all about. You know the feeling you got reading that story? Imagine actually feeling that in real life for yourself. This is what all that training and preparation is for. You've done the training, you've put in the work, you've made the sacrifices: now it's time to boss up and get that race medal.

In this chapter, I'll tackle all things race day, including managing your expectations, figuring out what gear to bring to the race, getting ready to race before the gun goes off, and racing after the gun goes off. We'll also tackle what to do after the race and how to deal with being DFL (dead fucking last), DNF (did not finish), or DNS (did not start). Finally I'll discuss how to deal with post-race depression. Are you ready? Let's go!

The Art of Picking a Race

Whether you're new to the sport or a running vet, selecting a race can be a daunting task. There are so many races to choose from, and once you start, it can be hard to stop. (After I ran that first 5K discussed in the cautionary tale, I wanted to run all of the races.)

After ten years of running races, I have come to the conclusion that race selection is more of an art than a science. Each race has multiple criteria (or colors) that make up the whole race experience (or the work of art). And as is true with a work of art, some of these criteria are in the eye of the beholder or the person running the race. Below is a list of my top ten criteria to consider when you're looking for a race to run.

1. Course Time Limit

Course time limits, sometimes called *course cutoff times*, are the times when the course officially closes and the organizers reopen the road or streets for regular traffic. Slower runners should definitely consider this when selecting a race. The description of the race on flyers, in advertisements, and on the race web page should clearly state the race's policy about time limits. Not only that, but that maximum finishing time should also be translated into a per-mile pace. If a participant does not meet that pace per mile, the race organizers should be clear about exactly what that means for the participant. Will you be removed from the race course? Will you have the option to move onto the sidewalk or side of the road where it is safe to continue? Will you get a finisher time? Do you still get a race medal if you did the distance but finished after the course limit? Will they still support you with hydration and race fuel after the cutoff? Is there a grace period?

Before signing up for a race, read its policies around these issues carefully. Ask yourself if they are up to your standards. Think about what your contingency plan would be if or when you fall behind the cutoff time.

If you are ever unsure about any aspect of a race, you can contact the race director for more information. Don't be shy about this. Answering questions is a part of their job!

A SMALL RANT ABOUT COURSE TIME LIMITS

This is an issue where running can get elitist. Go to any message board, forum, Facebook group, or the comments section of any post that talks about racing. You will find people shaming slow runners, saying these runners didn't earn their medals because they didn't make the cutoff, or complaining about the inconvenience of shutting down streets and paying security in order to cover longer cutoff times.

I say, what's an extra hour? Running is for everyone.

Regardless of the elitist assholes with their Twitter fingers, race times are being expanded and the community IS getting more inclusive. If you can't seem to find a race cutoff that suits you, don't be discouraged! Keep on looking!

2. Course Types

Race courses can be broken down into three types: loops, down-and-backs, and point-to-points. Each course type has its pros and cons when it comes to being a slower runner. I've listed some below, along with examples of races that fit the various categories.

Loops

Loop courses generally begin and end in the same place but follow a non-repeating route around the area. You could have one large loop or multiple smaller loops for your race. With a single large loop, you won't see the same thing twice, and you will start and end at the same place. Depending on how large the loop is, your family or friends who are watching the race could see you more than once along the course. Multiple loops can be both a gift and a curse because your spectators can see you multiple times, but you may get bored seeing the same thing over and over.

One cool thing about running a race that has multiple loops is that it can help you break the race into manageable chunks. The last benefit of a race with multiple loops is that race organizers may be more laid-back about the race cutoff.

Down-and-Backs

Down-and-back courses begin and end at the same location. They're similar to looped courses, but you follow one route to the halfway point before turning around and returning the same way you came. One of the benefits of running a down-and-back course is that you will have people around you for most of the race. At my first race, I was getting encouragement and high fives from the faster runners as they were on their way to the finish line.

One aspect of down-and-backs could be a pro or con depending on how you see it: having run the first half, you know exactly what to expect in the second half. This is good because you know what to expect, but you *are* seeing the same thing twice, which could cause you to be bored on the course.

Just as is true with the loop course, you can have multiple down-and-backs to complete a race. So you're going to experience some of the same pros and cons. Similar to loop courses, generally, down-and-backs tend to be lenient on the course cutoff time as well (your mileage will vary).

Point-to-Point

Point-to-point courses begin and end in different locations that are separated from each other by the distance of the race. Some of the world's most famous races are in this format, including the Boston and the New York City marathons. The cool thing about point-to-point courses is that you'll always have something new to look at throughout the race.

But there are also a few cons. Usually, point-to-point races begin earlier than others because you often have to be bused or take some type of race-provided transportation to the starting line. Additionally they generally have stricter cutoff times due to the nature of the course, which can span for miles across multiple cities, towns, or counties. This means that race support personnel, including those at hydration stations and the police, may leave sooner than you want them to. Also, the crowds will usually wane as you progress throughout the race. You'll never get cheers as loud or high fives from the faster runners—but the cheers you do get will mean so much more to you.

All these races have pros and cons. The only way to know which is best for you is to try 'em out.

3. Rolling Start vs. Wave Start

Another thing to consider is the way a race starts. With wave starts, you are put into a starting wave based on your predicted finish time. This typically means slower runners are at the back (hence the name *back-of-the-packer*), which can produce anxiety for some runners.

By contrast, with rolling starts, elite runners start first, and then there is a block of time when other runners can start the race. I personally love this type of start because if you're a slower runner, you can start at the beginning of the rolling start and give yourself a buffer from the time the course closes. I think it's a happy medium, and it gives everyone the opportunity to cross the finish line within the parameters of the course time limits.

4. Small vs. Large Races

When choosing a race, you'll want to weigh the benefits of running a smaller race versus running a larger race sponsored by a corporation. Smaller races may or may not have the personnel to support the back of the pack, but on the other hand, I've run smaller races that had a great "no runner left behind" attitude. Races organized by larger corporations may focus on efficiency and may have stricter rules. It's something to take into consideration as you shop for your ideal race.

5. Time of the Year

Typically racing is very seasonal. Most races happen in the spring or the fall. When selecting a race, you have to think about the time you're going to need to train for it. This means if you're aiming for a spring race, you're going to be training during the winter months. By contrast, if you're aiming for a fall race, this means that you're training through the dog days of summer.

Again, each season has its pros and cons, depending on where you live. You just need to weigh what works for you. Lastly, most races happen only once a year, so if there is a specific race that you want to run, there is no way of getting around training for it in a particular season. Decide and commit, or you'll be waiting another 365.

6. Walker-Friendly Races

There are races that call themselves walker-friendly, which means that they have longer course limits or no course limits at all. The benefit of this policy is not worrying if you're going to finish the race or not. These races are usually few and far between. But if you have one in your area or are willing to travel to participate in one, it may be right up your alley. Such races are a great way for newer, slower, or anxious runners to sample the race scene.

7. Medals and Race Swag

Many of us run races for the bling. Does a particular race have a medal or swag that's right up your alley? That might be a deciding factor for selecting that race. Many will share what the medals look like on their social media channels beforehand, so you can scope it out and see if you're interested in adding it to your collection. (It's going to be a collection, right?) Depending on what motivates you, you might also participate for the food treats afterward. One favorite race for many runners is the Thanksgiving turkey trot, which usually features slices of pumpkin pie at the end.

8. Race Start Time

I never thought about this until I learned about it the hard way. I signed up for a race and found out I had to be there at three A.M. so they could bus us to where we needed to be for a race start time of five A.M. Let my experience be a lesson to you: check the start times and see what time you need to be there. That could be a deciding factor. If I had known beforehand that I would have to be at that race so dang early, I wouldn't have signed up for it.

9. Entry and Travel Fees

If you're new to racing, let me be the first to tell you that running races isn't free. From $20 for a local run to hundreds of dollars to run in a major marathon, if your race roster is full, your bank account might take a hit. If you're on a tight budget, you may want to take this into consideration. It's up to you to determine if a race is worth your money, but there are certain criteria you can consider against the price. I personally look for a race medal (do I like it?), the swag offered, and the experience promised during the race. This is pretty rare, but some races also have scholarship entries for people who can't afford it—that's also an option to look into. Lastly, if you're traveling to a destination race, don't forget to factor in the expenses of travel, hotels, and meals because they do add up.

10. Reviews of the Race from Previous Runners

This is a BIG one. Word of mouth is still one the best ways to find races that support the back of the pack. Crowdsourcing other slow runners' experiences may influence your decision about certain races you're considering. A great place to start crowdsourcing race experiences is by asking members of the Slow AF Run Club (find us over at slowafrun club.com), as well as other groups dedicated to slow runners on social media.

Putting It All Together

After looking at the criteria, you can put them together like colors on a canvas to find a race that's suitable for your needs. What's important to you? And yes, I know I have given you lots to overthink about. Just remember that feeling good as you cross the finish line is the only thing that really matters.

Before Race Day

Now that you've selected a race, let's talk about preparing for the race. The days leading up to race day can feel overwhelming, full of pre-race jitters. Here are my best tips for preparing yourself for the big day.

Don't stay at the expo all day. A couple of days before the race, you'll need to go to the race expo and pick up your bib. For new runners, this is one of the biggest traps that you can get sucked into, so I'll be blunt about this: don't stay at the expo all day. Get your bib, ask the questions you need to ask, buy your souvenir, take your pictures, and go sit down somewhere. I'm serious. There's so much going on at race expos, between the vendors, the walking, and the people, that it will suck the energy right out of you. Your goal leading up to the race is to save as much energy as possible for the race itself.

Calm the fuck down. I don't know any other way to say this: calm the fuck down. Yes, I know it's easier said than done, but you've got to chill the hell out and calm the fuck down.

It's just a race; it's not the end of the world. There will be many more races to run, so calm the fuck down.

If you don't perform like you want to, you can sign up for another race at the same distance the following week, so calm the fuck down.

You've done the training, and the training is just the dress rehearsal for the real thing. You've done this over and over again. The only difference is that now you're doing it with more people, so calm the fuck down.

You have everything that you need already within you. Run your race and pace yourself, and you will do great, so *calm the fuck down.*

This is the pep talk that I give myself before every race. It works. It helps me get out of my head, because when all's said and done, none of this is that serious. EVERYONE gets pre-race jitters, pre-marathon zoomies, or whatever the kids are calling them these days. The journey is more important than the finish, and that's what I'm constantly refocusing on and forcing myself to remember.

Nothing new on race day. This is the golden rule of running. I don't know how many times I need to say this to the people I train. But please, PLEASE, **don't try anything new on race day.** I know you just bought new gear at the expo, but now is *not* the time to try anything new, please and thank you. Some potential consequences of running a race with new things that you haven't tried are injuries, gastrointestinal issues, blisters, sudden pit stops, and an overall unpleasant race experience. You've been warned, but I'm going to say it over and over until you remember.

Nothing new on race day. Nothing new on race day. Nothing new on race day. Nothing new on race day. Nothing new on race day times one hundred.

Carb loading and hydration. If you are running a shorter distance race, like a 1-miler, a 5K, or even a 10K, carb loading and extra hydration will probably not be necessary. But if you are running a longer race, this can be an important part of pre-race preparation. It's important to note: Hydrating and carb loading isn't something that happens the night before the race. It's something that happens three to five days before the race. Your body needs time to be able to process the food you eat to turn it into nutrients and store it in your muscles. Your body can process only so much at a given time, so you should be doing it over the days leading up to the race. Be sure to do some research and consult a professional to see whether carb-loading is right for your situation.

What Gear to Bring to a Race

In *theory*, you don't have to bring much because most races will provide you with water, a hydration mixture, and race fuel. However, most races cater to faster runners, so—depending on your pace, of course—there's always a chance you will get to a station and find it cleaned out. Furthermore, during your training season, you've probably become accustomed to a certain type of hydration mixture and race fuel, and nine times out of ten, the race you're running has a different fuel or hydration mix that may mess with your stomach. Keeping this in mind, support yourself during the race by bringing your own hydration and race fuel. That's what I usually do on race day.

What I bring to a race is similar to what I bring with me on my training runs. For 10Ks and under, I take water and a couple of race fuel packets. For half-marathons and beyond, I bring some sort of hydration pack,[1] and it's usually filled with the following things:

- My traveling pharmacy

---

[1] Be sure to check the rules of the race beforehand, because not all races allow hydration packs.

- Imodium/Pepto Bismol chewables
- Baby wipes or body wipes
- Aspirin or some type of pain reliever
- Band-Aids
- Fuel packets
- Salt tablets (just in case I'm losing more salt than I can put in)
- Anti-chafe lube
- Emergency cash
- My race fuel of choice
- Hydration mix
- Race maps
- Battery pack for my phone

On Race Day

Now it's time for what you've been doing all of this training and preparation for: actually running the damn race! Let's talk about a few things to make your racing experience more enjoyable.

Poop before the race. This is pretty self-explanatory. Pooping during a race is something runners love to do (yes, that is sarcasm), and if you haven't yet, you eventually will. I try my best not to poop in the Porta-Potties; the conditions in them are pretty horrendous during larger races. They often don't even have toilet paper (which is why I pack wet wipes). Also, I'm here to say that awful race toilets are a rite of passage you want to avoid as long as possible. If you got to go, then you got to go, but try your best to go before the race. You've been warned.

Continue to calm the fuck down. When the gun goes off, don't necessarily set out running like a bat out of hell. I know it can be tough to NOT get caught up with other people's pace. Don't do it! Settle in! Run YOUR race. You want to slowly ramp into your pace and groove. If you go out too fast, you risk getting injured, as well as not leaving enough gas in the tank to finish the race. If you've got a sports watch, use it to help you keep an eye on your time.

Pro Tip: If you're doing run/walk intervals, be sure to raise your hand when you are starting your walking interval so that people behind you will know to move around you, not to run you over. I learned this the hard way.

Don't take yourself too seriously. Listen, I know your first race can feel like (and IS) a big deal. Still, race day is a celebration of you! Have some fun with it! Talk to people, give out high fives, say thank you to the volunteers, read the signs, and take pictures. Enjoy. The. Struggle. This is what you did all this training for. Don't take yourself too seriously; enjoy the moment.

Pro Tip: Be sure to look for the race photographer as you are running so you can get some good pictures.

Have a strategy for race fueling and hydration. Most races will have some sort of hydration and fuel stations along the routes. You can add these into your race fueling strategy or ignore them and BYOG (bring your own gels).

For me, my race fueling and hydration strategy doesn't change from when I'm training. I've seen newer runners get full and sick after stopping and drinking at every station. I'm here to tell you that you don't need to drink at every stop. You've been following a specific plan during training; there's no reason to change it now (#NothingNewOnRaceDay).

No one is going to save you, aka manage your expectations. Beginner, nontraditional, slow, and fat runners: I'm going to get real with you for a second. Everything about racing is not gumdrops and unicorns. Here's the truth: no one, and I mean absolutely, positively no one, is going to save you out on that course. You got yourself out there, and it's your responsibility to get your butt to the finish line.

This is my mindset when it comes to running races. Being a slow, fat runner, I can tell you that no one is going to have mercy on you. Hell, the elitist runners might try to tear you down. I've had so many runners tell me to "lose weight and get faster." Nobody told me these next things that I'm going to tell you, and I believe it's my duty to forewarn you, since I've experienced them firsthand. If you're a slow, fat runner, I want you to be prepared:

- Be prepared for the race to not have shirts in your size.
- Be prepared not to have water at stations.
- Be prepared not to have race fuel.
- Be prepared to get lost because they took down the race signs.
- Be prepared to have a shitty experience.
- Be prepared for the race to run out of medals.
- Be prepared for the Porta-Potties to run out of toilet paper.

I want you to *stay* ready so you don't have to *get* ready. I'm telling you this because while racing can be a great experience, you have a higher chance of having to put up with some non-inclusive bullshit.

At one race, *all* the stuff in the list above happened to me. It sucked. It really sucked, but I got over it and kept racing because I love it. In spite of some shitty experiences, I refuse to be broken, and I'm going to keep talking about the bullshit that happens to the back of the pack until everyone is treated fairly.

If any of these things happen to you, let me be the first to say that I'm sorry, and it's fucked up. Be sure to share your experiences far and wide, as well as in the Slow AF Run Club (find us at slowafrunclub .com). Email the race director, letting them know how dissatisfied you are with your race experience. This is the only way to effect change. I'm with you all the way. We're together in the struggle.

Sure, I've had lots of GREAT experiences, too! But if I didn't warn you about some of the things that can happen, I would be doing you a disservice. You are powerful. You are a runner. **Now go out there with your head high. Give. Them. Hell. It's race day!**

Dealing with DFL, DNF, and DNS

You are bound to experience a DFL (dead fucking last), DNF (did not finish), or DNS (did not start) if you do this long enough. These hiccups don't feel good when they happen, but they are also not the end of the world.

LOTS of people DNF, not just back-of-the-packers. Look at the dropout rate at the men's marathon in the last 2021 Tokyo Olympics— it was substantial. If the elite runners can drop out of a race and move on with their life, why can't you do the same?

I've had all these things happen to me, and I've kept running strong for over ten years. The first point I want to make is not to take this too seriously. It's just a race; it may have been your goal race, but guess what? There will be other races to run. The second point is that again, it's all about the process over the results. Yes, this sounds cliché, but the thing I love most about running is the ritualistic nature of it. I focus on building the rituals, rather than worrying about the actual finish. Like for real. Finally, you *have* to listen to your body. There's *no* shame in choosing not to run or to stop running if you're in pain. You're not quitting; you're looking after your long-term health.

Remember, if you have any of these problems, you're going to be okay. It's like when you fell off your bike for the first time: it sucked. It hurt. Then you dusted yourself off and got back out there.

After the Race

Congratulations, you ran the race! You did the thing! You killed it! (I knew you would.)

After you cross the finish line, you may be overwhelmed by your emotions or other people's. You may feel disoriented as you try to find your family and get your race medal and snack. Here are a few tips to keep this part of the race smooth:

1. **Get your medal, take pictures, and get out of the way.** There's a lot going on at the finish line. Don't contribute to the bottleneck; get what you need and get out of the way. I do want to note that this is one of the benefits of being back of the pack. If the finish line is still up, you have a greater chance of good photo ops, since everyone has already finished! (Hell yeah!)

2. **Create a strategy for meeting with family and friends.** What's your estimated finish time? Where's your meeting point? What can they bring you? (This is mostly true for larger races.)

3. **Change clothes.** Nobody wants to be in sweaty wet clothes. Ask your friends or family to bring them, or if you're running alone, you can put them in gear check or in your car and pick them up after the race.

4. **Stay and cheer on other runners.** As a back-of-the-packer yourself, you know how much it means to receive cheers while you are crossing the finish line. Spread the love and cheer for runners coming in after you.

5. **Eat and hydrate.** The goal is to rehydrate and replenish your nutrients as quickly as possible. You might not be hungry, but getting some kind of nutrition is key—especially after distance races. The race will provide some food, but will it be enough? Maybe you can make a cool post-race tradition for yourself! Usually I have reservations at an Italian restaurant

after I run a race so that I can eat ALL the carbs. I also have a slice of carrot cake after every race. What will your post-run ritual be?

6. **Reflect and offer gratitude to your body.** This is pretty self-explanatory, but use this time to think about your race: what you enjoyed and what you would like to improve on. And while you are at it, express gratitude for the fact that your body is strong enough to do what you need it to do to get you across the finish line.

7. **Recover and plan for the next race.** Yes, your *next* race! Let's keep the momentum going!

Racing is one of the greatest pleasures of being a runner. Take my advice and you will experience highs and lows, make lifelong memories, and maybe change your life. However, just as racing can bring joy, the aftermath sometimes has unexpected consequences.

Post-race Depression, aka Post-race Blues

Post-race depression happens to plenty of runners. You spend so long training for something, you accomplish it, and then it's over. Months of work are brought to an end in one day. After I ran my first marathon in 2013, I got sad, really sad, and I lost interest in running.

I felt empty and a little hopeless. I found out there was a phrase for it: *post-race blues*. I'm here to tell you that you may experience this after finishing your race. I'm also here to tell you that it doesn't have to be that way. These are some of the things that I have done to combat it over the years.

Seek a therapist. One of the things that has done wonders for my running is talking to a therapist. Running can be intense! You impose pressure on yourself or suffer from anxiety or impostor syndrome or all of the above. Having an unbiased third party to help me talk through some of the things going through my head has been totally worth it. Also, finding a sports therapist is definitely a plus, because they know exactly what you are going through.

Sign up for more races. They say the best way to get over a race is to sign up for another race. One thing I've done is race stacking, which means having multiple races on my calendar within a particular season. This way, I'm not putting all my focus on one race; instead, it's on multiple races over a period of time. I've found this to be an excellent way to stay motivated to keep training because I don't want to lose my fitness before the other races.

> **Warning:** Do NOT put too many races close together because that's how you can get injured. Your body needs adequate rest between races. Of course this is going to be specific to you and your fitness level and the speed with which you recover after a race. You might be okay with back-to-back 5Ks or 10Ks, but when you jump up to half-marathons and full marathons, it will be different.

Give it time. Sometimes you need to let your body and mind recover, so taking time away from the sport is perfectly fine. I get it: training for a particular race is tiring, and sometimes you need a break. Running will be there when you're ready again, and while you're away, don't forget to cross-train to keep yourself active and fit (see chapter 8).

Wrapping It All Up

Despite these obstacles, I still love to run races. Why? Because crossing the finish line, no matter the challenges you face, always makes you more of an athlete, not less of one. You came and you conquered that shit! And that is something to be proud of. It's so rewarding and so worth it. I've met lifelong friends from races and traveled to places that I never would have traveled to because of running.

RACING QUESTIONS ASKED BY EVERY BEGINNER, NONTRADITIONAL, SLOW, OR FAT RUNNER

---

1. **What if the race description doesn't explain what happens if/when a runner falls behind the course limit?**

   Don't sign up for that race unless you are able to reach out to the race director and find out what exactly happens in that situation.

2. **I just bought some new shoes at the expo and I want to wear them at the race. Should I?**

   Absolutely not. Remember the mantra: nothing new on race day.

3. **Okay, but how long do I try something out before a race before it's considered not new (and wearable on race day)?**

   Every runner is a little bit different with their rituals. I personally wear something for up to three long runs before a race. That gives me a sense of how the product works for an extended amount of time that's similar to the race. But I usually tell my coaching clients that giving gear a test run two or three times before the race should be good. You just want to make sure that your body and/or the product reacts in the way that you want it to before the race.

4. **Besides the race cutoff time, what do you think is the most important thing when choosing a race?**

   It really depends. I like to use races as an excuse to travel the world, so I would personally say location. A close second would be if any of my running buddies are doing the same race; then I want to run it with them as well.

5. **Being around people makes me anxious, but I want to have a race to train for. Do you have any suggestions?**

    Actually, I do! There are virtual races, which you can do in the comfort of your favorite route, track, or park. Generally here's how it works: you sign up for the race, you do the distance and track it with your phone or GPS watch, you submit your information, and they send you a medal in the mail. If you are looking for virtual races, be sure to check out the Slow AF Run Club, as we put on multiple races a year.

6. **Do you have specific recommendations for how to decide if I shouldn't start a race on race day?**

    You need to trust your gut. If you don't feel mentally prepared or if you are injured or undertrained, don't do the race.

7. **How confident or practiced do I need to be at a given distance to sign up for a race? How many times should I have run that distance before race day?**

    Many training plans don't have you run the distance at all before race day. For example, when I ran my first marathon, my longest run up to that point was a 20-miler. So I lined up at the race not knowing what would happen to me after mile 20, but I completed the race! The idea is that if you did at least 80 percent of the training plan, you'll be able to finish the race distance.

CHAPTER 7

Recovery Matters

Cautionary Tale: A Running Streak Right into Injury

In 2014, a few months after my first marathon, I got into a bad car accident that took me away from running for a good year and a half. When I finally got the okay to run again, I was bound and determined to make up for the time that I missed. I wanted to expedite my training so I could get back to where I was before the car accident. Spoiler alert: *This was an absolutely terrible idea.*

I went from not running at all to deciding to take on a winter running challenge to run every day from Halloween until New Year's Day. During this run streak, my goal was to run at least 1 mile every day (again, this was a terrible idea). At first everything was fine. I started at 1 mile a day for a couple of weeks without issue. I was feeling so good that I started to increase my miles. One mile a day became two, two became three, and next thing I knew, I was running seven or eight miles a day (which, once more, was a terrible idea).

As I progressed through my quest to gain back everything that I'd lost with the car accident, I started to feel some tenderness in my knee (warning sign number one). *No worries*, I thought. *I'll take an aspirin before I run.* Knee tenderness evolved into tightness in my hips and IT bands (warning sign number two). *No worries, I'll just stretch a little bit . . .*

I kept running day after day, week after week, ignoring the warning signs until the day after Christmas. I was tired and dazed, but I was still determined to finish the challenge. My body was achy all over, but I had only a few days left. I rolled out of bed to do my daily run. As soon as my foot touched the floor and I put weight on it to stand up, I felt something sharp in the heel and the arch of my foot. A little voice in the back of my head was telling me to take the day off.

I've been going strong for close to two months. What's a day of rest? No! I need to prove to myself that I can do this.

So I went running that day. The next day when I woke up, the pain was a little worse, but I continued to run anyway. The next day it was a little worse. I kept on this cycle until the last day of the challenge, New Year's Eve. When I got out of bed, I could barely put any weight on that leg. As I hobbled to put on clothes and struggled to put on my shoes, that little voice advised me to take the day off. I responded: *I'm almost done.*

The voice suggested taking the mileage down and doing just one mile. *No, I must finish what I started.* So I went out and attempted yet another 8-mile run. Two miles into this I started to feel a burning sensation in my heel. Eventually the burning sensation got so bad that I had to stop running and hobble over to the shoulder of the road to sit on a tree stump. Yes, the same tree stump from the cautionary tale in chapter 4. I called Char and told her to come get me. As I sat in the car, I knew that I had done more harm than good. I waited a few days for it to get better, but it didn't.

I went to the doctor, and it was confirmed that I had run my way into plantar fasciitis and Achilles tendinitis. I had done the exact thing that I was running from. I ended up injured and had to sit out for months, go to physical therapy, have shock wave therapy, prolotherapy, platelet-rich plasma injections, MRIs, X-rays—just about every procedure that could be done short of surgery. It took me close to another year to be back to 100 percent, and by then I had lost everything and had to start back over again. It was a hell of a lesson to learn.

Most new runners (including me during that time) think that if they're not running every day, then they're not runners, and that is so far from the truth. Taking breaks and planning for recovery make you more of an athlete than charging forward recklessly with your health.

Recovering properly is important because it decreases the chances of injury and gets you back on the road as quickly as possible. I don't want you to follow in my footsteps, as that will only lead to your getting injured. So in this chapter, we'll be discussing why recovery matters, what tactics for recovery you should consider, and how to stay injury-free (after weekly running sessions AND after major races).

I will describe how I was able to run four marathons in a single year while weighing over 300 pounds—injury-free! If you don't get anything else from this chapter, I want you to take away that we need rest and recovery time, and if we don't take them, our bodies will start to break down. That's when you get sloppy and get injured. I'll complete the chapter (you guessed it!) by tackling recovery questions asked by every beginner, nontraditional, slow, or fat runner.

Why Recovery Matters

The famous running coach Jack Daniels (yes, that's his name—no relation to the whiskey) once said, "Rest is a part of training, it is not avoidance of training." Recovery needs to be a part of your ritual as an athlete. I'm not just talking about taking a day off once or twice a week or getting an occasional massage, though both of these are effective strategies. Recovery is just as important as running and training. It should be a part of your culture, your identity as an athlete. Being in tune with your body is important. This is something that we all need. **Running + Rest = Running Success.**

Recovery is the period when our muscles repair themselves. But recovery by itself is not enough, because if you don't run, there's no way to add the stress to your body necessary to trigger the hormone to promote muscle growth.

Thanks to social media, hustle culture and the workaholic mentality have become the toxic mainstays of our lives. Everything is all about hustling hard. What happened to the adage "work hard, play hard, recover hard"? (Or did I just make that up?) I'm constantly challenging myself to work hard and recover harder.

Being an athlete involves rituals. Start thinking about your rituals after training runs and after races. You should be deliberate about these routines regardless of whether you're feeling good or not. Make recovery a part of the ritual. Now let's dive in a little deeper and talk about three types of recovery: passive recovery, active recovery, and mindset recovery.

Passive Recovery

When we think about rest or recovery, passive recovery is what most people think of. During passive recovery, the body stays completely at rest. Passive recovery is important and beneficial if you're very tired, either mentally or physically, after exercising and you need to recharge your batteries, or even when you're injured or in pain. Here are a few tips to work this important kind of recovery into your routine.

> **Put your feet up and chill out.** Think sitting on your butt with your feet up while watching Netflix! I love to rest my feet in my recovery boots (see page 143 for more on compression boots) and watch sports documentaries (I like watching

sports docs because watching someone go through the struggle and make it to the other side is inspiring) or sitcoms like *The Bernie Mac Show*, *Martin*, *The Fresh Prince*, or *The Office*. I also enjoy playing board games or video games (I'm unstoppable at UNO! and Mario Kart). Of course, you need to know when to take a break from screens and give your body some deep rest. Which brings me to my next point.

Sleep. When you sleep, your body repairs and restores itself and recovers, which is why getting adequate rest is important. Sleep rebuilds our brains and bodies by releasing hormones such as growth hormones and testosterone and allows us to stay focused throughout the day. According to the Centers for Disease Control and Prevention, 35.2 percent of all adults in the United States report sleeping on average for less than 7 hours per night. Furthermore, 62 percent of adults around the world say they don't sleep as well as they'd like. Not meeting your sleep needs can affect way more than your running. It can cause a lack of energy, trouble remembering things, a reduced attention span, slowed thinking, a reduced sex drive, poor decision-making, irritability, daytime sleepiness, and other mood changes.

According to the American Academy of Sleep Medicine, 88 percent of American adults reportedly also lose sleep due to binge-watching. If you're a part of that group, we need to have a larger conversation about your priorities. Is that TV show that you can watch later most important, or do you want to get a good night's rest to perform better when you are running the next day? Let's hope it's option B.

To get good sleep, you need to do some assessment. What is your sleep ritual? How do you wind down for the day? For me, it's important that my bedroom feel like a cave. I have blackout curtains, and I put tape on anything that has an LED light so it's completely dark. I keep my cell phone in a different room. I take CBD edibles or a tincture to help make me drowsy. I set a 30-minute time limit on TV, and when the timer goes off, I practice the 4-7-8 breathing exercise[1] until I fall asleep.

Figure out what rituals work best for you, because you simply cannot perform at the highest level without great sleep. Obviously this will involve some trial and error. The best way to start is to get your phone out of your bedroom and give yourself some limits on TV time before bed. Then think about what relaxes you: a scent, a sound, or a vibe in your room? Establish a good sleep routine and hygiene.

Eat. Rehydrate + refuel = recovery. Eating and drinking after a run will increase your energy, boost your immune system, and help you get the most out of each day and training session. Recovery will improve your hormone response, decrease inflammation, and improve tissue quality, thus decreasing the number of overuse injuries you may experience. We discussed this at length in chapter 4, but I'll say it again: you're fueling more than your performance. You're fueling your recovery. What you eat on your days off matters just as much as what you eat on your running days.

By understanding these key elements of passive rest, you are well on your way to becoming a running recovery master.

Active Recovery

Active recovery, or what I sometimes like to call shakeout recovery, is when you participate in low-intensity activity either after your

---

[1] To do the 4-7-8 breathing technique, inhale through your nose for a count of four. Next, hold your breath for a count of seven. Then exhale completely through your mouth, making a *whoosh* sound, for a count of eight. (Purse your lips if it helps.) This completes one cycle; repeat for a total of four cycles.

workout or on your rest day. I like to call it shakeout recovery because it feels like you're literally shaking out the cobwebs of stiffness and soreness. Active recovery can help reduce soreness and tightness after a run or workout. It can also help improve your performance in the long run.

According to a 2018 study, some of the benefits of active recovery include reduced lactic acid buildup in the muscles, increased blood flow to muscle tissue, removing metabolic waste from the muscles, and reduced muscle tears and pain.

Active recovery days should include activities different from your usual workout, so pick something other than running. You also shouldn't be working at maximum effort. You should go slow and not push yourself too hard. Remember, the main goal is to shake out the cobwebs of soreness, not necessarily to get aerobic benefit from the activity. When doing active recovery, you shouldn't be breathing hard or even break a sweat. In the day or two after a strenuous workout, you can still participate in active recovery. Your active recovery repertoire can include a variety of methods and exercises, each of which can have different benefits.

Examples of active recovery exercises include:

- Restorative yoga or light stretching
- Light resistance training
- Walking
- Swimming
- Foam rolling
- Cycling

The possibilities are endless with active recovery. The main thing is to raise your heart rate just a bit to help you stay loose. You may find that you feel less tight or sore, or even that you have more energy to exercise after active recovery. If you're injured, in pain, or very fatigued, you should be doing passive recovery instead.

Mindset Recovery

Just as your body needs to recover, your mind needs to recover as well. This is something that is often completely ignored when it comes to running, but I'm here to tell you that mental fatigue is a real thing, especially when you're going through a three- to four-month training season.

Running can bring up tough shit and skeletons in your closet. It can bring up raw emotions, including doubt and anxiety. Remember in chapter 6 when I talked about seeing a therapist? This is one of the reasons why. Good recovery includes making space for your mental health, because running isn't a cure-all.

Again, running is 90 percent mental and 10 percent physical. You have to make sure you are taking care of that muscle in between your ears. That is where grit and determination is built, and sometimes you need a mental break. Nobody can be in go mode all the time.

Practice Other Hobbies

Often athletes get so wrapped up in a particular training block or goal that they lose sight of why they're training so hard. This can lead to burnout. Mental breaks during your training, when you focus on other hobbies/life stuff for a bit, allow you the time to look objectively at what's important to you and why it is that you're training. These breaks are also the perfect opportunity to evaluate your current plan and set goals for the future.

During this time, focus your attention on other aspects of your life. Don't let your whole life become about running! Do other stuff. SERIOUSLY! The all-or-nothing mentality will not work; it will only hurt you. It's so easy to become obsessed with running. If you let it, running will consume you and become all that you think about, read about, and research.

My advice: Find other things to do! It may be a project you've been meaning to get to, family time, or another hobby that you've wanted to try. These extracurricular activities will keep you engaged and feeling productive, and ultimately you'll be more refreshed to train for your primary sport. Here are some activities that have helped me with burnout and given my mind a break:

- Yoga
- Family time
- Meditation
- Journaling
- Playing video games
- Watching my favorite TV show
- Whatever else I like to do to recharge my batteries that doesn't include running or working out

Hopefully this will spark some ideas for you. Remember, don't overthink this. The goal is to focus your attention on aspects of your life other than running. Recharge the batteries often because you want to be in the sport of running as long as possible. This is a lifelong journey!

Recovery Professionals

As running becomes an important part of your life, you'll want to start thinking about your recovery team. As the old saying goes, it takes a village to raise a runner! You don't need to have all the professionals below on your team when you first get going. However, eventually working with them will ensure you can stay healthy and in your running shoes for as long as possible.

Here are some trained practitioners you can consult about your running health:

- General practitioner
- Chiropractor
- Physical therapist
- Acupuncturist
- Podiatrist
- Massage therapist
- Athletic trainer
- Cryotherapist
- Sports nutritionist/dietitian
- Other running-specific sports medicine doctors

I go see my general practitioner before every race season and get a physical exam and blood work done. This is more for a baseline to help me as I progress throughout the season. A few times a year I'll get my blood work done just to make sure I'm not deficient in anything.

As I get deep into the season, I'll start to see a physical therapist for prehab, which involves therapy-based movements and exercises in order to avoid injury or decrease pain. It is known as a proactive approach and can address deficits in strength, stability, range of motion, balance, and overall joint function. This is all a precaution so that I can work on imbalances before they cause injuries. When I'm feeling extra tense, I go see a massage therapist. I especially like massages after a race or a long, tough run. Of course, running is my passion AND my work, so this definitely isn't something everyone needs to worry about. It's about finding out what works for you.

My Recovery Toolbox

Over the years, I've picked up a lot of tools from physical therapy, the gym, or just experience. If a practitioner uses something on me and my body responds well to it, I'm buying it for myself. Here's a list to consider for your own recovery toolbox. Again, it's all about finding what works for you.

- **Foam roller, massage ball, lacrosse ball, golf ball.** Ever heard the phrase *hurts so good*? Yeah, they were probably talking about these tools. Each of them can help roll out tight spots in your muscles.

- **Graston tool.** If a foam roller hurts so good, then a Graston tool hurts like hell. These may look like brass knuckles or torture implements, but really, they are another instrument that helps break up scar tissue or muscle knots. (Apparently.)

- **Massage gun.** If you don't want to hurt as bad on a foam roller and want some convenience, then try a massage gun. You won't get as deep a massage, but it's a good tool to have on hand and you can use it while watching Netflix.

- **Compression recovery boots.** Have you ever dreamed about what it's like to be the Michelin Man? Trying stepping into some recovery boots. (Seriously, google these things.) They use air to create compression on your legs, restricting and then allowing blood flow. These boots are touted as giving you fresher legs after use.

- **Ice bath.** Exactly what it sounds like. After a long run, fill a bathtub with cold AF ice and water and sit in it. Soak your legs for 10 to 15 minutes, but no more than that. (You probably won't need encouragement to get out!) The belief is that this helps remove metabolic waste from the muscles and speeds up recovery because the cold constricts your blood vessels and improves blood flow.

- **TENS machine.** A transcutaneous electrical nerve stimulation (TENS) machine is a small, battery-operated device that is for pain relief, involving the use of a mild electrical current to trick your brain into recognizing the current versus the pain. You're literally shocking the pain away.

- **Cupping set.** Remember the 2016 Rio Olympics when Michael Phelps looked like he got attacked by an octopus? Well, that's because he was being treated through cupping. This is an ancient Chinese medical practice that uses small suction cups to bring blood to the skin. Cupping is touted as a method to improve circulation and treat pain.

You can add any or all of these to your personal recovery toolbox, but I recommend getting advice and instruction from a well-trained professional before you get into serious do-it-yourself territory.

Putting It All Together: My Recovery Rituals

Now that we've talked about recovery methods, it's time to put it all together. Below you'll find my typical routine, as well as notes on the specifics of how I incorporate the types of recovery into my schedule. As I said, this is my ritual; you need to create your own ritual that works for you and your schedule.

Martinus's Weekly Schedule During Running Season

Monday	Tuesday	Wednesday	Thursday	Friday	Saturday	Sunday
Passive Recovery	Run + Cross-Train Optional	Cross-Train + Active Recovery	Run	Passive Recovery + Mindset Recovery	Long Run	Active Recovery + Cross-Train Optional

Now you might be thinking, *Martinus, I'm a beginner. How do I work in recovery?* I got you! Below you'll find a schedule that is a little bit more suited for beginners.

Example of a Recovery Schedule

Monday	Tuesday	Wednesday	Thursday	Friday	Saturday	Sunday
Run	Active Recovery + Cross-Train Optional	Run	Cross-Train	Passive Recovery	Long Run	Passive Recovery + Cross-Train Optional

After every run:

- Stretch.
- Foam-roll.
- Use recovery boots.

After every three to four weeks of training, it's recovery week:

- My mileage and intensity drop significantly for this week. I'll get a massage and check in with appropriate members of my recovery team (mainly a physical therapist or a general practitioner to get blood work).

After every race:

- Get carrot cake (very important!).
- Refuel and rehydrate.
- Put CBD salve on any aches and pains.
- Use recovery boots.
- Take a nap.
- Refuel and rehydrate again.
- Get a massage the next day.
- Follow up with my physical therapist or the appropriate member of my recovery team if I'm having any aches in the following week.

Recovery is non-negotiable for a successful athlete (this includes you). I challenge you to include one of each of these types of recovery days in your running schedule. You'll soon reap the benefits of a well-balanced body and mind (after you finish foam-rolling and cursing me out).

RECOVERY QUESTIONS ASKED BY EVERY BEGINNER, NONTRADITIONAL, SLOW, OR FAT RUNNER

1. How many rest days can I take before I lose fitness?

    It depends on where you are physically. For example, if you ran a marathon, then took two weeks off, that wouldn't necessarily affect you. However, taking two weeks off in your first month of running might.

2. How often do I need to see a health professional?

    This is something that you and your healthcare provider should discuss. I'm not here to provide medical advice, just to let you know there are options for you.

3. What if I can't make myself stop and recover? What if I feel like I'm not doing enough?

    Seek a therapist. Something in your past may make you think you don't deserve rest or that there's no choice but to be stuck in hustle culture. I'll say this: If you do too much, too soon, and don't rest, you will get injured. Take care of your body, yo.

4. When do I resume my regular training after a race?

    It depends on how you're feeling, and when your next race is. I personally take about a week to ten days off from running before hopping back into my regularly scheduled training.

For more inspiration and examples on how to add recovery into your repertoire, check out chapter 7 of your Slow AF Run Club Bonus Companion Course, which you can get access to at slowafrunclub .com/course.

CHAPTER 8

Cross-Train or Die! (Or Risk Injury)

Cautionary Tale: Dead Ass! No, Really, Dead Ass Syndrome

Remember in chapter 7 how I told you that I had a running streak from Halloween to New Year's Day one year and ignored every single warning sign my body was urgently trying to send me? Let's talk about that some more.

After that injury, I finally got the green light to run again, and I was super stoked about it. The thing that I didn't tell you in chapter 7 is that I had an entry into the New York City Marathon that year and ultimately had to defer it because of, you know, injuries.

One year later, I was injury free, and the deferral was going to expire. So I had two options. Option 1: Do the responsible thing, let the deferral expire, and try my luck with the lottery for the New York City Marathon for the following year. (Who knew if lightning would strike again, but that would be the responsible thing to do, since I had just come off an injury.) Option 2: I train for and run the New York City Marathon. It was January, so if I started right away, I'd have roughly eleven months to train for it. I could slowly ramp up into things, and by the summer I could fully swing into training. So I did what any person who has never run the New York City Marathon does. I started training for it.

Training after an injury is by far the most nerve-racking experience ever. You feel like you can never get into a groove and find the flow state because you're hyperaware of every . . . single . . . thing your body is doing. Every step, every stride, every creak your bones make—you're overly aware because you're wondering, "Is this it? Am I injured again?"

A few months went by, and eventually I found my stride. Running felt effortless again, but then another wrench was thrown into the mix. Char told me that she got a new job and that we would have to move from New England to the San Francisco Bay Area. This made a tough training season even tougher. Moving from one coast to the other, finding a new job, and scouting out places to train made for a very tough time adjusting to everything.

As I settled into my new life in the Bay Area, my training started to suffer. My new job required me to work long days, and it became a struggle to fit running in. But somehow I did. I started running super early in the morning, like at four or five A.M., or cut my daily mileage in half and did half in the morning and half at night. I got in the training but didn't have time for much else. Then it happened again. I started to get nagging discomfort and tightness in my legs. On one run it would be my calves; on the next it would be my hamstrings or my quads. It was all over the place. This time I heeded the warning signs and made an appointment with a physical therapist. As we were going over her assessment, I told her that I was a runner and filled her in about my issues, my previous injury, and my goal to run the New York City Marathon. She nodded her head and took notes on her laptop. Then she asked me to lie back and do a glute bridge on one leg and then do the same on the other side. She asked me if I lifted or did any cross-training or strength training other than running. Nope. Not since I moved there. I was just running at that point. I had no room in my schedule for anything else.

"Hmm," she said. "Well, you, sir, have dead butt syndrome."

Say what?

Gluteal amnesia, which is common in runners; they develop it when they have imbalances and cause other muscles to overwork, which keeps the glutes from firing correctly.

"So you're saying that I have a dead ass?"

"Pretty much."

"Well, how do we revive my ass? Because the marathon is calling."

"Well, you need to work on glute activation and overall strength."

That's when I knew I needed to rethink my approach to running. Again! Yes, I was running consistently, but that was all I was doing. You have to do other things to make sure your health as a runner is sound. When I was first injured, I thought I learned that all my aches, pains, and discomfort came from not resting enough or giving my body time to recover. This time around, I learned it was due to muscle imbalance resulting from a lack of cross-training and strength training. Weak muscle here, tight muscles there, non-firing muscle everywhere. Dead ass. I had dead ass syndrome.

Most new runners think that if they're running consistently that's the only thing they need to do, but this is far from the truth. I want you all to repeat after me: *If I don't make time to cross-train, I will be making time for physical therapy and doctor visits.* Unless you have a crush on your physical therapist or doctor and want to see them on a weekly to biweekly basis, you'd better be making time to cross-train. Get it? Got it? Good!

In this chapter, we'll explore other important elements in running that aren't running at all: cross-training and injury prevention. I'll break down cardio and strength cross-training. I'll share my cross-training routine, and I'll explain what to do when you get injured and how not to beat yourself up during an injury. I'll complete the chapter by tackling cross-training and injury prevention questions asked by every beginner, nontraditional, slow, or fat runner.

Ready? Let's get into it!

What the Fuck Is Cross-Training?

Cross-training (sometimes written as XT in training plans) is any physical activity that isn't running. We're talking about cycling, yoga, weightlifting, swimming, hiking, and even getting your groove on in a dance class (or your living room). These are all cross-training, and cross-training should be an important part of your running routine. I know what you're saying: *Martinus, some of these activities are considered active recovery as well.* Yes, that is true. The difference between cross-training and active recovery is that you are looking to get the cardio benefit from cross-training, whereas during active recovery, you're not necessarily doing the activity for a workout or cardiovascular benefit but to stay loose and limber.

Cross-training:

- Helps prevent injury.
- Gives you mental and physical rest from running.
- Builds up muscle groups running may not target.
- Helps you maximize your running efficiency.
- Helps maintain or even improve your cardiovascular fitness.

In short, it's non-running that makes you better at running. It's key. Important. Unskippable.

The Two Types of Cross-Training

Cardio Cross-Training. Cardio cross-training is anything that
gets your heart pumping. Just like running, it can improve
your cardiovascular endurance. Swimming and cycling
(indoors on a stationary bike or out in the real world) are two
of my favorite types. These two activities are non-weight-
bearing exercises, which means they give your body a break
from pounding the pavement. Again, literally anything can
be cardio cross-training, and you don't necessarily have to be
in the gym to do it.

You could also do specific cross-training activities
that mimic running form and improve the cardiorespira-
tory system. These include aqua running, cross-country
skiing, elliptical machines, stair-steppers, walking/
hiking, swimming, cycling, in-line skating, and ice
skating.

Strength Cross-Training. Strength cross-training is also crucial
for any runner. It's a great tool for injury prevention because
it helps improve the strength and durability of your muscles,
bones, and joints. This is really important. Runners have high
injury rates—like, hella high. It's been reported that almost
half (46 percent) of all recreational runners incur injuries
regardless of age. Furthermore, if you have had a previous
injury, you are twice as likely to get a running-related injury as a runner with no previous injury. Cross-training is
one way to stop injury in its tracks. Yoga, weightlifting, and
even calisthenics are a few ways you can help yourself by
building muscle mass and improving structural weakness in
the body. Running works only a certain set of muscles. Thus,
you will start to have muscle imbalances if you do nothing
but run.

> **Remember:** If you don't make time for cross-training, strength training, and stretching, you'll be making time for physical therapy and running rehab.

Recovery is also important, and it relates to cross-training; you can't have one without the other. See chapter 7 for a refresher on passive and active recovery.

How Often Should You Cross-Train?

In a perfect world, a trained-up runner should be running three to four days a week, cross-training two to three days a week, and resting for at least one day. I know at times we aren't always trained up, and the last time that I checked, none of us lives in a fairy tale. So, if you're adjusting and struggling to add cross-training into your routine, try adding just **one day** per week. Work up to two days when you think you have the time. This is key for maximizing its benefits.

While writing this book, I was training for and ran the Boston Marathon. (There is a whole other book in that journey, believe me.) Again, this was my training schedule.

Monday	Tuesday	Wednesday	Thursday	Friday	Saturday	Sunday
Passive Recovery	Run + Cross-Train Optional	Cross-Train + Active Recovery	Run	Passive Recovery + Mindset Recovery	Long Run	Active Recovery (or Shakeout Run) + Cross-Train Optional

You might notice something in there—something very important. My schedule includes the word *optional*. Training schedules aren't written in stone, and some days you need the option to do things if you feel like you can or not to do them if you don't feel like you can. You'll also see that I stack my gym/cross-training days with days that I have a shakeout run. I like to add it there; that way I can have two days of passive recovery instead of one. I also like to note that this is a training that I developed with additional assistance from my running coach. (Yes, even running coaches have running coaches. It's so meta.) Everything that you see here is not a one-size-fits-all type of thing. Just as was true with trying on running shoes and everything else, you're going to have to customize it for yourself: your schedule, your physical ability, and the distance that you're training for.

Also, when you're thinking about cross-training, look at your weaknesses and address them with other activities. (I personally like one cross-training day to be a moderate-to-high-intensity CrossFit type of strength workout and the other cross-training day to be low-to-moderate-intensity strength training or something like cycling or swimming.) The main thing is being aware of your imbalances and working to improve them. Tight muscles? Focus on loosening them up. Dead ass? Work on glute activation. These are the times to work on your weaknesses to make you a better runner. Gentle workouts like mobility-enhancing yoga or moving meditations are a perfect choice for a rest day.

Your At-Home DIY Cross-Training Routine

At this point, maybe you're saying, "Martinus! I have no idea about how to work out or where to begin when it comes to cross-training. Please help!" No worries, homie! I got you! You don't need a gym membership or special equipment to get started with cross-training. When you're just starting out, your body weight and some dumbbells will be enough to challenge you.

Below are four cross-training circuits you can do at home in your living room, basement, backyard, or wherever. For starters, add them in once or twice a week on the days that you don't run or days that you have lighter runs. I don't suggest cross-training on your long run days. For instructions on how to do these moves properly, see below. I've also included modifications for the exercises as well so you can modify them down (make the exercises easier to perform) or modify them up (make the exercises harder to perform) depending on your needs.

Also, you'll notice that I provide a range for the repetitions and sets. But these numbers are not set in stone. They are just to give an idea of your options: you can do low reps and low sets, low reps and high sets, high reps and high sets, or high reps and low sets. If you're starting out, I recommend starting with the lower end of reps and sets for the first couple of weeks just so your body can get used to the exercises and you can increase reps and sets as needed. Also, pay attention to your fatigue level. When I say fatigue level, I mean that if you had a tough run on the day in question or the day before, your body will already be tired, so you will need to adjust the reps and sets as needed.

> **Remember:** Recovery and cross-training work together. I find that if I put just one number down even though I've told my clients that it's a range and that they can scale down if needed, they still go for the set and rep that I've given them, even if they are toast from a previous workout.

Also, be sure to rotate the circuits. Do an upper-body and lower-body routine each week, and don't do the same circuit twice in the same week. I've added a table below to give you some ideas on how to mix up the circuits using my schedule as an example. None of this is rigid, so adjust any part of it to make it work for you.

Eight-Week Cross-Training Schedule

	Monday	Tuesday	Wednesday	Thursday	Friday	Saturday	Sunday
Week 1	Run	Active Recovery + Leg Day Circuit B Optional	Run	Upper/ Core Day Circuit A	Passive Recovery	Long Run	Passive Recovery + Leg Day Circuit A Optional
Week 2	Run	Active Recovery + Upper/ Core Day Circuit A Optional	Run	Leg Day Circuit B	Passive Recovery	Long Run	Passive Recovery + Upper/ Core Day Circuit B Optional
Week 3	Run	Active Recovery + Leg Day Circuit B Optional	Run	Upper/ Core Day Circuit A	Passive Recovery	Long Run	Passive Recovery + Leg Day Circuit A Optional
Week 4	Run	Active Recovery + Upper/ Core Day Circuit B Optional	Run	Leg Day Circuit B	Passive Recovery	Long Run	Passive Recovery + Upper/ Core Day Circuit A Optional
Week 5	Run	Active Recovery + Leg Day Circuit A Optional	Run	Upper/ Core Day Circuit B	Passive Recovery	Long Run	Passive Recovery + Leg Day Circuit B Optional
Week 6	Run	Active Recovery + Upper/ Core Day Circuit B Optional	Run	Leg Day Circuit A	Passive Recovery	Long Run	Passive Recovery + Upper/ Core Day Circuit A Optional
Week 7	Run	Active Recovery + Leg Day Circuit A Optional	Run	Upper/ Core Day Circuit B	Passive Recovery	Long Run	Passive Recovery + Leg Day Circuit A Optional

	Monday	Tuesday	Wednesday	Thursday	Friday	Saturday	Sunday
Week 8	Run	Active Recovery + Upper/ Core Day Circuit A Optional	Run	Leg Day Circuit B	Passive Recovery	Long Run	Passive Recovery + Upper/ Core Day Circuit B Optional

Ways to Complete the Circuits

There are two ways that you can complete the circuits. You could complete the first exercise for the full number of sets before moving to the next exercise, or you could complete the first exercise, then move on to the second, then the third, until you're done with the circuit, then repeat the circuit once you're done with the desired sets that you wanted to do. Either way is completely fine. However, I would recommend that you take a 1- to 2-minute break between each exercise and at least a 3- to 4-minute break after completing a circuit (all the exercises in a block).

For some of these exercises, I ask you to take an athletic stance. Here's what that looks like: Stand with your feet shoulder-width apart, your hips and knees slightly bent. Look straight ahead and keep your chest open. Lock your body into position by engaging your core, which involves drawing your belly button into your spine. (I always imagine that someone is about to punch me in the gut!)

If you are looking for pictures and videos about how to do these exercises, check out chapter 8 of the Slow AF Run Club Bonus Companion Course at slowafrunclub.com/course. Then you'll be ready to roll.

UPPER/CORE DAY CIRCUITS

Upper/Core Day Circuit A

1. Push-ups (3–15 reps, 3–5 sets based on fatigue level)
2. Standing biceps curls (10–15 reps, 3–5 sets based on fatigue level)

3. Triceps kickbacks (10–15 reps, 3–5 sets based on fatigue level)
4. Bent-over rows (10–15 reps, 3–5 sets based on fatigue level)
5. Dead bug (10–15 reps, 3–5 sets based on fatigue level)
6. Plank (20–90 seconds, 3–5 sets)

1. **Push-ups**

    Muscles targeted: chest, shoulders, upper and middle back, biceps, triceps, core, hamstrings, quads

    How to do it: Get down on all fours, placing your hands firmly on the ground, slightly wider than your shoulders. Straighten your arms and legs. Engage your core by drawing your belly button into the spine to lock your body into position. Lower your body, keeping your back flat and your eyes focused about 3 feet in front of you to keep a neutral neck, until your chest nearly touches the floor (inhale going down). Pause, then push yourself back up (exhale going up).

    Modifications

    Modify it down

    Do your push-ups standing upright, pushing off the wall.

    Drop to your knees and do a push-up from that position, keeping your back flat as you drop down and return back up.

    Modify it up

    Add weight by putting a couple of pairs of shoes in a backpack and wear the backpack while you are doing push-ups.

    Put your feet on a chair, couch, or box and do push-ups in that position.

2. **Standing biceps curls**

    Muscles targeted: biceps, forearm flexors

    How to do it: Start by standing in your athletic stance (see page 156). Keeping your elbows tight at your sides, hold a dumbbell in each hand. Let your arms relax down at the sides of your body, palms facing forward. Keeping your upper arms still and your shoulders relaxed, bend at the elbow and lift

the weights so that the dumbbells approach your shoulders.
Your elbows should stay tucked in close to your ribs (exhale
while lifting the weight). Once your hands are near your
shoulders, pause for a second, squeezing the biceps muscle at
the top. Slowly lower the weights to the starting position
(inhale while lowering the weights).

Modifications

Modify it down

Sit on a bench instead of standing.

Use lighter weights.

*Use resistance bands instead of weights. Step on the band
handle, hold the other handle in your hand on the same
side, and perform the exercise. Switch and do the other
side.*

Modify it up

Use heavier weights.

3. **Triceps kickbacks**

   Muscles targeted: triceps

   How to do it: Start by standing in your athletic stance
   (see page 156). Hold a weight in each hand. Lean forward
   from the waist, bringing your torso almost parallel to the
   floor, and keeping your back straight. Bend your arms
   90 degrees at the elbow so your triceps are aligned with your
   back and your biceps are perpendicular to the floor. On the
   exhale, hinge at the elbow and straighten your arm, lifting
   the dumbbell up and back. Your triceps should stay still; only
   your lower arm and hand move. When your arm is straight,
   pause, then on the inhale, return the weights to the starting
   position.

   ### Modifications

   Modify it down

   Perform the exercise with lighter weights.

Do one arm at a time, placing your free hand on a bench for
support.

Modify it up

Increase the weight of the dumbbells.

Pause for 1 to 2 seconds at the top of the extension.

4. **Bent-over rows**

   Muscles targeted: upper and middle back, shoulders, biceps, core

   How to do it: Start by standing in an athletic stance (see page 156). Hinge at the waist at a 45-degree angle and push your hips back. Hold the dumbbells with your palms facing the floor (overhand grip). On the exhale, pull the dumbbells up under your chest as far as possible. Imagine there's a lemon between your shoulder blades, and try to squeeze the juice out of it as you pull the weights to your sides. Pause for 1 to 2 seconds, and then on the inhale, slowly lower the dumbbells back to the starting position.

   Modifications

   Modify it down

   Do a single-arm row, placing your free hand on a bench for
   support.

   Use lighter weights.

   Modify it up

   Use heavier weights.

5. **Dead bug**

   Muscles targeted: core

   How to do it: Lie on your back with your legs in tabletop position above your hips, arms reaching toward the sky with your palms facing in and back pressed to the ground. Keep your core engaged by drawing your belly button into the spine to lock your body into position. On the exhale, slowly lower your right arm and left leg until they're out straight just above the floor. On the inhale, bring them back to the starting position. Repeat using the opposite arm and leg. This completes one repetition.

Modifications
Modify it down
Lower just one limb at a time instead of moving opposing arms and legs simultaneously. This means you extend your right arm by itself. After you bring it back to center, extend your left leg. After you bring your left leg back to center, do the same thing with your left arm and right leg.

Modify it up
Hold a lightweight dumbbell in each hand as you perform the arm and leg extensions.

Hold a medicine ball with both hands. Extend both arms and both legs at the same time and return them to center together.

6. **Plank**

   Muscles targeted: core, back, shoulders, glutes

   How to do it: Assume a push-up position, with your feet together and your body straight from head to heels. Make sure your wrists are directly beneath your shoulders.

   Squeeze your glutes and engage your core by drawing your belly button into your spine to lock your body into position. Hold the position. Don't hold your breath. Breathe!

   To do a forearm plank, assume a push-up position but place your weight on your forearms instead of your hands, with your elbows directly beneath your shoulders. Then follow the rest of the instructions above.

   ### Modifications
   #### Modify it down
   Perform the plank while you are on your knees. Keep your back straight.

Modify it up
Lift one leg or arm up. You could also hold the opposite leg and
arm up.

Upper/Core Day Circuit B

1. Bird dog (10–15 reps, 3–5 sets based on fatigue level)
2. Superman/back extension (10–15 reps, 3–5 sets based on fatigue level)
3. Dumbbell chest press (10–15 reps, 3–5 sets based on fatigue level)
4. Dumbbell side raises (10–15 reps, 3–5 sets based on fatigue level)
5. Dumbbell shoulder press (10–15 reps, 3–5 sets based on fatigue level)
6. Upright rows (10–15 reps, 3–5 sets based on fatigue level)

1. **Bird dog**
    Muscles targeted: core, lower back, glutes, quads
    How to do it: Get down on all fours, with your hands directly below your shoulders and your knees directly below your hips. This is the starting position. Keep your back flat and your core engaged by drawing your belly button into the spine to lock your body into position. On the exhale, simultaneously extend your left leg straight behind you and your right arm straight in front of you. To help your balance and stability, imagine that the hand and knee that remain on the ground are actually trying to pull the floor apart underneath you.
    Pause for 1 to 2 seconds, and on the inhale, return to the starting position. Repeat with your right leg and left arm. This completes one repetition.
    Modifications
    Modify it down

Raise just one limb at a time instead of two simultaneously. Don't lift your limbs as high.

Modify it up

Place a resistance band handle around one foot and hold the other handle in your opposite hand. Extend your banded arm in front of you and your banded leg behind you.

2. **Superman/back extension**

    Muscles targeted: core, lower back, glutes, hamstrings

    How to do it: Lie facedown on the ground. Fully extend your arms in front of you. On the exhale, simultaneously raise your arms, legs, and chest off the floor while squeezing your lower back. Hold the position for 3 to 5 seconds. Don't hold your breath. Slowly lower your arms, legs, and chest back to the floor while inhaling.

    ### Modifications

    ### Modify it down

    Do an alternating superman: Lift your opposite arm and leg at the same time and hold for 3 to 5 seconds. Slowly lower your arm and leg and repeat on the other side.

    Lie facedown with your arms out in front of you, the tips of your fingers pressed against the floor. Instead of lifting your arms, press hard on the tips of your fingers and lift forward and up through your neck and shoulders. Simultaneously stretch your legs back and up as high as you can go.

    ### Modify it up

    Perform the exercise holding a medicine ball, dumbbell, or kettlebell.

3. **Dumbbell chest press**

    Muscles targeted: chest, shoulders

    How to do it: Lie on your back on the ground with your knees bent and a dumbbell in each hand, your bent arms resting beside your chest, with your elbows on the ground, palms facing your knees. On the exhale, use your chest to push the dumbbells up. Lock your arms at the top of the lift and squeeze your chest, hold for a second, and then on the inhale, lower the weights slowly.

Pro Tip: Lowering the weights should take about twice as long as raising them.

Modifications
Modify it down
Perform the exercise using lighter weights.

Use a resistance band instead of weights. Place the band crosswise under you, grasp one handle of the band in each hand, and then press up and lower the handles.

Modify it up
Use heavier weights.

Hover your feet above the ground a few inches while you are pressing.

Raise to a glute bridge while pressing up.

4. **Dumbbell side raises**

   Muscles targeted: shoulders, upper back

   How to do it: Start by standing in your athletic stance (see page 156). Hold a pair of dumbbells with palms facing inward and let them hang at your sides. On the exhale, raise your arms out to the sides until they are at shoulder level. Pause at the top for 1 to 3 seconds. Then on the inhale, slowly lower the weights back to the starting position.

   ### Modifications
   #### Modify it down
   Perform the exercise one side at a time.

   Use lighter weights.

Use a resistance band instead of weights. Stand on the middle of the band, grasp one handle in each hand, and perform the exercise.

Sit instead of standing.

Modify it up

Use heavier weights.

Stand on one leg while performing the exercise (but pay attention to that core form!).

5. **Dumbbell shoulder press**

   Muscles targeted: shoulders, upper back, core

   How to do it: Stand in your athletic stance (see page 156). Hold a set of dumbbells at shoulder height, with both arms bent, elbows at 90 degrees, and palms facing forward. On the exhale, press the dumbbells overhead until your arms are fully extended. Pause, and then on the inhale, slowly lower the weights back to the starting position.

   ### Modifications

   ### Modify it down

   Use lighter weights.

   Sit instead of standing.

   Perform the exercise one arm at a time.

   Use one dumbbell with both hands.

   ### Modify it up

   Use heavier weights.

   Do a squat between reps.

6. **Upright rows**

   Muscles targeted: shoulders, upper back, core

   How to do it: Start by standing in your athletic stance (see page 156). Grab a pair of dumbbells in an overhand grip and hold the weights in front of your thighs with your palms facing your body. Keeping the weights as close to your body as possible, on the exhale, pull the dumbbells up toward your chest. Your elbows should remain flared out during the movement. When the dumbbells are at chest level (not at your chin), pause for 1 to 2 seconds. Then on the inhale, lower the dumbbells back to the starting position.

Modifications

Modify it down

Use lighter weights.

Use a resistance band instead of weights. Stand on the middle of the band, grasp one handle in each hand, and perform the exercise.

Modify it up

Use heavier weights.

Do a squat between reps.

LEG DAY CIRCUITS

Leg Day Circuit A

1. Clamshells (10–25 reps, 3–5 sets based on fatigue level)
2. Glute bridges (10–25 reps, 3–5 sets based on fatigue level)
3. Air squats (5–15 reps, 3–5 sets based on fatigue level)
4. Walking lunges (5–15 reps, 3–5 sets based on fatigue level)
5. Single-leg Romanian deadlifts (5–15 reps, 3–5 sets based on fatigue level)
6. Calf raises (10–25 reps, 3–5 sets based on fatigue level)

1. **Clamshells**

   Muscles targeted: glutes, hips

   How to do it: Lie on your right side with your feet and hips stacked, your knees bent 90 degrees, and your head resting on your right arm. Draw your knees in toward your body until your feet are in line with your butt. Place your left hand on your left hip to ensure it doesn't tilt backward. This is your starting position. On the exhale, keep your core engaged by drawing your belly button into the spine to lock your body into position. Keeping your feet together, raise your left knee as far as you can without rotating your hip or lifting your right knee off the floor. Hold for 1 to 3 seconds, squeezing your glutes at the top of the move. On the inhale, slowly lower your left knee to the starting position. After you're done with the reps, repeat the exercise on the other side to complete one set.

Modifications

Modify it up

Loop a resistance band around both thighs, just above your knees, and perform the exercise.

2. **Glute bridges**

Muscles targeted: glutes, quads, hamstrings, core

How to do it: Lie on your back on the floor with your knees bent and your feet flat on the floor. Place your arms out to your sides at a 45-degree angle to your body. Engage your core by drawing your belly button into the spine to lock your body into position. On the exhale, press your feet on the ground and lift your hips so your body forms a straight line from your shoulders to your knees, while squeezing your glutes. Pause with your hips in the air for 3 to 5 seconds. On the inhale, lower your body back to the starting position.

Modifications

Modify it up

Hold a dumbbell above your hips while you perform the exercise.

Loop a resistance band around your thighs above the knee to perform the exercise.

Raise one foot off the ground while you perform the exercise.

Perform a chest press while you perform the exercise.

3. **Air squats**

     Muscles targeted: calves, quads, hamstrings, glutes, core

     How to do it: Stand in your athletic stance (see page 156).
On the inhale, flex your knees and hips and sit back, leading
with your hips and butt. As you squat, keep your head and
chest up and push your knees out. Continue down as far as
you can. On the exhale, quickly push your heels through the
ground until you return to a standing position.

     Modifications

     Modify it down

     Don't go down as far.

     Use a chair or bench and sit in the chair, then stand up.

     Modify it up

     *Hold and/or pulse for 5 to 10 seconds at the bottom of the
          squat.*

     Add a hop after performing the exercise.

     *Loop a resistance band around the thighs just above the knees
          and perform the exercise.*

     *Hold a dumbbell in each hand, or one with both hands, and
          perform the exercise.*

     Add a lateral leg raise after performing the exercise.

     Add a calf raise after performing the exercise.

4. **Walking lunges**

     Muscles targeted: calves, quads, hamstrings, glutes, core

     How to do it: Start by standing in your athletic stance
(see page 156). On the inhale, step forward with one foot,
bending the knees to drop your hips. Descend until your rear
knee nearly touches the floor. On the exhale, drive through
the heel of your lead foot and straighten both knees to raise
yourself back upright into the starting position. Step forward
with your opposite foot, repeating the lunge with the opposite leg. This completes one repetition.

Modifications

Modify it down

Only go halfway down when performing the lunge.

Modify it up

Carry dumbbells while performing the exercise.

Hold and/or pulse for 5 to 10 seconds at the bottom of the lunge.

Add a hop after performing the exercise.

5. **Single-leg Romanian deadlifts**

    Muscles targeted: hamstrings, glutes, ankles, core

    How to do it: Start by standing in your athletic stance (see page 156). Stand on one leg. On the inhale, keeping your knee slightly bent, bend at the hip, rotating your torso forward while simultaneously extending your free leg behind you for balance until your body is parallel to the floor. Keep your body in a straight line. On the exhale, return to the upright position. Repeat the reps for this same leg, then switch to the other leg.

    Modifications

    Modify it down

    Instead of extending your free leg behind you for balance, keep it on the ground but kickstand it behind you.

    Hold on to a chair or the wall when performing the exercise.

    Modify it up

    Hold dumbbells or kettlebells in your hands while performing the exercise.

6. **Calf raises**

    Muscles targeted: calves

    How to do it: Stand straight and tall, with your hands on your hips, your core engaged, and the balls of your feet firmly planted on the ground. On the exhale, raise your heels as high as you can so that you're on your toes. Hold the position for 1 to 3 seconds, and on the inhale, lower your heels back to the ground.

Modifications

Modify it down

Hold on to a chair or wall for extra balance while performing the exercise.

Modify it up

Hold a dumbbell in each of your hands while performing the exercise.

Perform the exercise while standing on one leg.

Perform the exercise while standing on the edge of a step, your heels hanging slightly over the edge.

Add a hop at the top of the rep.

Leg Day Circuit B

1. Fire hydrants (10–25 reps, 3–5 sets based on fatigue level)
2. Donkey kicks (10–25 reps, 3–5 sets based on fatigue level)
3. Lateral lunges (5–15 reps, 3–5 sets based on fatigue level)
4. Romanian dumbbell deadlifts (5–15 reps, 3–5 sets based on fatigue level)
5. Sumo squats (5–15 reps, 3–5 sets based on fatigue level)
6. Wall sit (20–90 seconds, 3–5 sets)

1. **Fire hydrants**

   Muscles targeted: glutes

   How to do it: Get down on all fours, hands shoulder-width apart, knees under your hips, elbows slightly bent. Your core should be engaged by drawing your belly button into the spine to lock your body into position. Your back should be straight and parallel to the ground, not arched or swayed downward. On the exhale, keeping your knee bent, raise your right leg out to the side until it's parallel to the ground. Hold for 1 to 3 seconds, and on the inhale, slowly return to the initial position. Repeat on the left side. This completes one repetition.

Modifications

Modify it up

Loop a resistance band around your legs above your knees and perform the exercise.

Instead of being on all fours, hover your knees off the ground and then perform the exercise.

2. **Donkey kicks**

   Muscles targeted: glutes, lower back, core

   How to do it: Get down on all fours, hands shoulder-width apart, knees under your hips, elbows slightly bent. Your core should be engaged by drawing your belly button into the spine to lock your body into position. Your back should be straight and parallel to the ground, not arched or swayed downward. On the exhale, keeping your knee bent and foot flexed, lift one leg up behind you until your thigh is in line with your body and your foot is parallel to the ceiling. On the inhale, lower your leg back down. Repeat with the other leg. This completes one repetition.

   ### Modifications

   Modify it up

   Extend straight foward the arm that is opposite your raised leg.

   Instead of being on all fours, hover your knees off the ground and then perform the exercise.

3. **Lateral lunges**

   Muscles targeted: glutes, hamstrings, quads

   How to do it: Start by standing in your athletic stance (see page 156). On the inhale, take a slow step to the left side. Keep your toes pointed forward. Allow your knee and hips to bend, moving your weight down and to the left in a side lunge. Pause for 1 to 3 seconds, and then on the exhale, straighten the bent leg to return to a standing position, transitioning into a lunge on the opposite side. This completes one repetition.

Modifications

Modify it down

Lunge about halfway down.

Modify it up

Hold a pair of dumbbells while performing the exercise.

Hold and/or pulse for 5 to 10 seconds at the bottom of the lunge.

4. **Romanian dumbbell deadlifts**

    Muscles targeted: glutes, quads, hamstrings, lower back, traps

    How to do it: Start by standing in your athletic stance (see page 156). Hold a pair of dumbbells in front of you with an overhand grip, palms facing the body. On the inhale, hinge forward at your hips, keeping your knees slightly bent, lowering the dumbbells to the ground without allowing your back to round. On the exhale, lift back to the standing position. Keep your head in line with the rest of your body and avoid arching your neck.

    ### Modifications

    Modify it down

    Perform the exercise with no weights.

    Modify it up

    Perform the exercise with heavier weights.

5. **Sumo squats**

    Muscles targeted: calves, quads, hamstrings, glutes, hips, core

    How to do it: Start by standing in your athletic stance (see page 156). Hold a pair of dumbbells in front of you with an overhand grip, palms facing the body. Stand

with your feet 3 to 4 feet apart and your toes slightly turned
out. On the inhale, bend your knees and sit back with your
hips into a squat, keeping your head and chest up. On the
exhale, push through your heels into the ground to stand
back up.

Modifications

Modify it down

Perform the exercise with no weights.

Don't squat down as deep.

*Perform the exercise with both hands holding one dumbbell
instead of two.*

Modify it up

Perform the exercise with heavier weights.

6. **Wall sit**

Muscles targeted: quads, glutes, hamstrings,
calves

How to do it: Start by standing with your back against a
wall or a stable hard surface. Slide your back down the wall
until your hips and knees bend at a 90-degree angle. Keep
your shoulders, upper back, and the back of your head
against the wall. Both feet should be flat on the ground
with your weight evenly distributed. Hold for the desired
duration.

Modifications

Modify it down

*Don't squat as deep; aim for a 45-degree angle at the hips
rather than a 90-degree angle.*

Modify it up

Perform the exercise holding dumbbells.

*Perform biceps curls, lat raises, or shoulder presses during the
wall sit.*

Perform the exercise on one leg.

These are just a handful of exercises that you can do on your cross-training days. Don't think of these exercises as the be-all and end-all; remember that these are just some general exercises to get you started, and they aren't personalized to your needs as an athlete, because everyone is different. If you are looking for something specific for your needs, I would recommend engaging a personal trainer. If you're looking for more accountability to cross-train, be sure to join the Slow AF Run Club (find us at slowafrunclub.com). We have a biweekly virtual class that you can join in on!

Injury and Pain Management

The goal of adding cross-training to your plate is to improve your running and to prevent injury. Don't let the tech T-shirts, social media posts, and Strava stats fool you: runners are getting injured all the time, and they shouldn't be.

LEGAL AF DISCLAIMER

I'm not a doctor, and I don't play one on TV, so take all this advice with the appropriate grain of salt. If something hurts, take a couple of days off from running and get it checked by a doctor. Pushing through pain will only make things worse and could cause permanent damage.

When Not to Run

When you're in the middle of a solid running routine, it's hard to skip runs. I get it—I've been there. Pretty much all the runners I know (including me) have tried to test the limits of the body by trying to sneak in a run when they shouldn't have (or sometimes a whole run streak's worth of running when I should have listened to my body).

Pro Tip: If the pain is sharp, stabbing, or in a joint, it's likely bad. If it's dull, achy, sore, and in a muscle, it's likely good and okay to move on. (Note that I said "likely" and not "for sure.")

If you're feeling some pain, here's how to know when it's time to skip a run:

- The pain is present when you walk.
- The pain feels concentrated in one area.
- The pain gets worse while running.
- If the pain escalates slowly as you're running, STOP RUNNING!
- If the pain hits once you're warmed up, STOP RUNNING!

If you're experiencing any of these symptoms, don't go running or walking; don't pass Go and collect $200. Got it?

Here are some signs you might be okay to run:

- Your pain occurs at the outset and decreases as you move.
- Your pain occurs briefly and disappears.
- You're pretty sure it's delayed onset muscle soreness (DOMS).

DOMS is the pain and stiffness felt in muscles several hours or days after unusual or strenuous exercise. The soreness is felt most strongly 24 to 72 hours after the exercise.

The Difference Between Soreness and Pain

When you're dealing with a possible injury, the temptation to push yourself can be very real. When this happens, it can be important to understand the difference between pain and muscle soreness.

The chart below highlights key differences between muscle soreness and pain.

	Muscle Soreness	Pain
Type of discomfort	Tender when touched; tired or burning feeling while exercising; minimal dull, tight, and achy feeling at rest	Ache; sharp pain at rest or when exercising
Onset	During exercise or 24 to 72 hours after activity	During exercise or within 24 hours of activity
Duration	2 to 3 days	May linger if not addressed
Location	Muscles	Muscles, joints, or bones
Improves with	Stretching after movement, and/or more movement, with appropriate rest and recovery	Ice, rest, and more movement, except in cases of significant injury
Worsens with	Sitting still	Continued activity after appropriate rest and recovery
Appropriate action	Get moving again after appropriate rest and recovery, but consider a different activity before resuming the activity that led to soreness	Consult with medical professional if pain is extreme or lasts more than 1 to 2 weeks

A Note on Spatial Awareness

When you first start running, it can bring on a lot of new and interesting aches, pains, and feelings of discomfort. Lots of people tune out of their bodies while running to help manage some of that. They let their thoughts wander or turn up music. Here's the thing: tuning into your body while you run and staying aware of your surroundings is also key for injury prevention. This is called spatial awareness. You're less likely to trip over a rock on a trail or a sudden curb if you're locked in on your surroundings. You're more likely to notice the twinge or tug of a muscle if you're paying attention to every step. Do your best to stay tuned in, and you'll reap the benefits.

What to Do When You Get Injured

What to do when you get injured? Shit, homie, it happens to everyone, but it won't happen to you, right?! Because you're going to be listening to your body and working on correcting your weaknesses and imbalances. Just know that injuries happen to everyone, there's no shame in it, but also follow this to the letter and listen to your body and you'll be fine. Don't beat yourself up; allow yourself the time to heal. Running ain't going anywhere, and it will be here when you get back. Understand that it's a process. You got this. Heal up and come back stronger.

CROSS-TRAINING AND INJURY PREVENTION QUESTIONS ASKED BY EVERY BEGINNER, NONTRADITIONAL, SLOW, OR FAT RUNNER

1. How much cross-training is too much?

    If you're feeling out of it (meaning fatigue or lethargy), then you're probably doing too much.

2. Is it possible to run a marathon without cross-training? Why is it so important?

    You can do whatever you want. But from my experience and from the experience of the people who I have trained, you want to cross-train. Overall, it makes you a better runner, and the consequences of not cross-training can be injury and sitting on the sidelines. You'll have muscle imbalances that cause other muscles to become overworked, resulting in an overuse injury. Do you want that? Because I don't want that for you. It's best to throw some type of cross-training into your schedule.

3. How many days a week is a good amount to aim for when cross-training?

    If you're new, I would recommend starting with one day of cross-training and then building up from there. If you're in the middle of training for a race, I don't suggest doing it more than three days a week. You want to make sure you're giving your body adequate time to rest as well. See my schedule above on page 152. That's a pretty packed week, and I wouldn't want to add anything else because you need time to rest and live the rest of your life. That stuff is important, too.

4. Can I cross-train and run on the same day?

Yes, you can do this—with two caveats. Don't do it on your long run day because you want to give your body adequate time to recover from your long run, and do your run *before* you work out.

5. What are your thoughts on cross-training on rest days?

Rest days are a rest from running; it doesn't mean you rest from being an athlete. So go for it. As long as you have additional passive rest days on your calendar, then you should be good to go.

6. I like to lift heavy and am starting as a runner. Can I lift heavy while I train for long distances?

Yes, but you can't serve two masters. You need to decide what is going to be your primary mode of movement and what is going to be secondary. For example, during the wintertime I rarely run, so I can focus on lifting heavy and getting stronger. When it's time to train for a race, I still lift but it's not heavy nor is the aim to get stronger or to increase my max weight. It's about keeping those accessory muscles strong, as well as spending the training session working on any imbalances that I may have. Another way to put it is, whatever you're looking to dial in and improve is what you want to do first because you're gonna have the most fuel and energy for that. So if it's running or any other sports-specific thing and you want to dial in your skills in that sport, you're gonna want to do that training before you do weight training. If you're looking to build strength, then you're going to want to do weight training before your skills training, or even running, for that matter. Also, you're going to want to have time between the two (running and weight training), because you're going need to refuel before doing the other.

CHAPTER 9

Goals for Days (and Months and Years)

Cautionary Tale: 300 Pounds and Goalless

People often ask me how I've stayed motivated throughout the ten years I've been running. They see me on social media and think that I'm up early every day before sunrise to crush 10 miles, drink a gallon of kale juice, do 2 hours of yoga, write in my journal, and then get back out to run another 10 miles—all before nine A.M. But that's far from the truth. I wasn't always the 300-pound-marathon-running badass that I am today. (You've read enough of my cautionary tales to know that by now!) There have been times when I wasn't motivated or crushing any goals. Hell, there have been times when I didn't even have goals. I haven't always been the podcast host, Slow AF Run Club founder, and *Runner's World* cover model. Once upon a time I was just Martinus.

It was the year after I ran the New York City Marathon. Yes, I FINALLY brought my ass back to life and crossed the finish line in 2018. I was ready for more, so I put my name in the lotteries for all the Abbott World Marathon Majors. These are the six largest marathons in the world: New York City, London, Berlin, Tokyo, Chicago, and Boston. I was sure that I had a good chance of getting into at least one of these races and I couldn't wait. See, after running the New York City Marathon I was hooked and wanted to train only if I was running one of the World Majors again. My motivation was tied to these big races, and I was counting on them for inspiration to get laced up again.

If you don't know, these races are large (for example, the 2019 New York City marathon had 53,627 runners crossing the finish line), so that's why you need a lottery to participate in them. On the lottery days for World Major races, runners who have their names drawn always take it to social media. The lotteries for these races take place over a span of a few months, and that year I was waiting on every single one of them.

The draw for Tokyo was first. I saw a friend's post saying that he got in. I eagerly checked my email: nothing, not even in the spam folder. (Although I did receive an email from a Nigerian prince saying he wanted to give me a million dollars.) I went back to my inbox and refreshed the browser: nope, nothing. Again. Nothing. On social media it seemed that all my friends had gotten that magical, mythical, life-changing email.

Then, just as I was about to give up hope, I checked my inbox one last time. There it was: the email I'd been waiting for all day. But, when I opened it, it didn't look like the email all my friends had posted on social media. "We regret to inform you . . ." I sighed deeply, shook my head, closed the window, and went back on social media to congratulate all my friends.

Despite the Tokyo setback, I was still hopeful; there were four more race lotteries. I shouldn't have been so optimistic. Remember the cautionary tale in chapter 8? My hope that lightning would strike twice and I'd get drawn in the New York City Marathon lottery again? Well, that particular year, I didn't get a cloud, thunder, or even a spark of static electricity. As the months passed, the rejection emails piled in. After each one, I stayed hopeful; surely I would get into one, right?

Finally, the last rejection email arrived. I hung my head as a single tear ran down my cheek. I had been so sure I would get into one of the World Major marathons that I hadn't put any other races on my calendar. I scrambled to find other popular races to sign up for, but they were all sold out. Damn it!

As the months went by without a goal in sight, I lost momentum. I had nothing to look forward to, nothing to work for. My running routine was sporadic, inconsistent. I moved less and less as the weeks went by. I felt terrible about this and about myself.

Why can't I stay motivated to run?

That's how I learned something very important about myself: if I wasn't racing, I wasn't running—at all. I knew I needed to rethink my approach. Yes, again!

From the outside, I may look like an inspired and motivated individual, but that isn't the case—not exactly, anyway. I work at it.

Why does it always seem like motivation and success are natural? Like some people have it, some don't? Maybe you think something is wrong with you because you can't stay inspired or motivated. But I'm here to tell you that just isn't true. Here's the problem: motivation is fleeting. It's situational, it's emotional, and it's not what brings long-term success. When the doctor called me fat, I was motivated to prove him wrong. I ran that first marathon, and more after that.

However, over the years, his words lost their sting. I started to forget his name; truthfully, everything about that situation stopped hitting me as it did when I first started running. The anger and defiance that had motivated me burned away after 30 many miles. A good kick-start, but not enough fuel in the long term. I often found myself in one of two cycles: the "fits and spurts" cycle, in which I frequently started and quit; or the "depression and emptiness" cycle, in which I put a lot of energy into a goal, reached it, and then felt a sense of emptiness or despair after the success and happiness of achievement faded. This is what happens when you put all your time and energy into completing one thing—once that thing is over, you're not sure what to do next. You get lost. This happens to everyone!

Am I naturally motivated? No. I'm not even a natural runner. I wasn't a runner as a kid; hell, in high school, I hated running and failed the 1-mile test. But I put my work in and I came to love it; it became part of my identity.

Yet somehow, after running a race, I couldn't maintain my habit of running. This led me to ask myself: What do I do when I'm not feeling great? How do I run when I'm not motivated or inspired to run? I went to therapy, I read, I journaled, and I figured out what made me tick. Now I'm here to share.

I learned that staying power comes from values, goals, processes, and rituals. In this chapter, I'll pull the curtain back and share what has helped me keep running over many years. Heads-up: This chapter is part reading and part workbook. It will require you to do some participation and reflection to get the most out of it. So grab a pencil and get ready! Let's get into it.

Defining Values: What the Heck Are They?

Values are the fundamental beliefs and guiding principles that inform your behaviors and actions. Think of values as your internal compass, your North Star, your internal GPS. They let you know if you're moving in the right direction in life.

Values are not the same as goals. A value is like heading east: you can go in that direction, but you can never really reach east because it's not a destination. Goals are an attainable destination, something you can achieve. Living your values is an ongoing process.

For example, if you want to be a loving, caring parent, that is a value—an ongoing process. If you stop doing loving and caring things, then you are no longer a loving and caring parent; you are no longer living by that value. In contrast, if you want to have a kid, that's a goal—you can achieve that and cross it off your list. Once you have a kid, you're a parent. Running the New York City Marathon is a goal. Once you've run it, your goal is achieved. On the other hand, fully applying yourself as an athlete and runner is an example of a value—an ongoing process.

Another distinction between values and goals is that values generate goals. One value can generate an infinite number of goals.

Values may also fall under different domains, such as partnership and intimate relationships, parenting, family relationships, social relationships, career, education and training, recreation, spirituality, citizenship/community, or health/fitness/physical well-being. For this chapter, we'll stay focused on values related to health/fitness/physical well-being. (I'm a run coach, not a life coach!) At the same time, the material in this chapter could help you define your values and set goals in all the areas of your life.

Determining Your Values

As a runner and a human being, you need to know what your values are. That's essential to making your life meaningful. If you don't know what you value, you don't know where you're going! Your values reflect what is most important to you: what kind of person you want to be, what you consider significant and meaningful, and what you want to stand for in your life. Your values provide direction for your life and motivate you to make important changes.

Here's a simple exercise to help you start defining your values. Please take a few minutes to write out your answers below. We're going to get a little morbid for a second. Imagine you're at your own funeral. There are flowers and sad music, and your family and friends are crying because you've gone to be with your ancestors. Take a second to imagine it.

It's the part of the service when people talk about you. What are they saying? What do you want them to say? Imagine the conversation drifts toward your health and fitness. Take a minute to write down what these people would say about you.

Example: "Martinus never let his weight get in the way of living the life he wanted. He overcame every obstacle . . . Hell, he ran a marathon when he weighed 300 pounds and was on the cover of *Runner's World!*"

_____

_____

_____

_____

_____

_____

_____

_____

_____

_____

_____

Keep imagining your funeral. Now think about these questions: What's important to you? Who do you aspire to be? What relationship do you want to have with running and movement in general? If you weren't driven by emotions and fear, who would you be? If you had no negative emotions or fear around running, physical activity, and movement, then what would you do with your body? Write these down, too.

_____

_____

_____

_____

_____

_____

_____

_____

_____

Then finish the following sentences:

When it comes to my health, fitness, and physical well-being, I spend too much time worrying about _____

_____

_____

When it comes to my health, fitness, and physical well-being, I spend too little time doing things like _____

_____

_____

When it comes to my health, fitness, and physical well-being, if I could go back in time, I would _____

_____

_____

Take a second to read this over to yourself. These sentences point to your values around health and fitness.

Now that you've identified some of your health and fitness values, let's take this exercise a step further. You've probably written a lot above, and it's probably all over the place, and that's okay. Now it's time to condense and rewrite your health and fitness value (or values) into a one sentence affirmation. Write one sentence for each value. Write these values in the present tense.

Examples: "I move joyfully!" "I am an accomplished runner."

_____

_____

_____

_____

_____

_____

_____

_____

_____

_____

_____

_____

How did it go? For most people, this exercise is quite an eye-opener. It often highlights the difference between what we value and what we're actually doing. Now, don't let these values just sit here in these pages. Take them with you into the world. Write them on Post-it Notes and stick them in places where you will see them every dang day. Make them into affirmations. Constantly remind yourself what you stand for and are striving for. Read your values as many times as you can, every day, until they become your truth.

Setting SMARTY Goals

Now that you have identified your values, you know what really matters to you. You've calibrated your internal compass, and you know which direction you need to go. Now what? Don't worry, there's still work to be done. Things don't happen just because you've identified your values. Change happens when you take action using your values as your compass. One way to start taking action is by creating SMARTY goals based on your values. SMARTY goals are a twist on the better-known SMART goals. This powerful acronym is a road map to setting great goals that you can actually reach. A great goal should be:

Specific: Goals should be clear and specific (e.g., not "I want to run farther," but "I want to run a 5K" or "I want to build from my 10-miler to a half-marathon").

Measurable: Goals should have concrete trackables (e.g., "I will run three times a week").

Attainable: Goals should be realistic. You're not going to go from jogging around the block to running a marathon in a month. What is an achievable short-term goal? What about long term? (For example, "I want to add cross-training into my running once a week.")

Relevant: Goals should be important to you; if they don't matter, you won't feel driven to pursue them. Does it seem worthwhile to you? Is it the right time to tackle this challenge?

Time-Sensitive: Goals should include a time frame or a deadline to help you focus and dig in. You can set goals for a week, a month, three months, six months, or any time frame you like. As long as your time frame has a fixed end point, you're good. (Just don't use time points that are too far away. This is about your short-term goals, not your five-year plan.)

Your Big Why: This is my personal addition to SMART goals. Why do you want to achieve this goal? Why is it important? Your why is your overarching reason for going after the goal. When you struggle with motivation, this is the fuel for your inner fire. When the honeymoon phase is over and you just don't feel motivated, when your family is less supportive than they used to be, your big why is the only thing that will keep you going. A good why is powerful. Are you emotionally tied to it? Does it really matter to you? Can you lean on it when the going gets tough? Every time you set a goal, you need a why to go with it.

Using the SMARTY method to set goals that are guided by your values is a great way to start on your way to personal success. This is key; without your values and goals, you could end up in the "fits and spurts" cycle and/or the "depression and emptiness" cycle that I mentioned earlier.

Now that you know what SMARTY goals are, take one of the health and fitness values you identified earlier and create a few SMARTY goals based on that value.

Health and fitness value: _____

_____

_____

_____

_____

SMARTY Goal #1: _____

_____

_____

_____

_____

SMARTY Goal #2: _____

_____

_____

_____

_____

SMARTY Goal #3: _____

_____

_____

_____

_____

SMARTY Goal #4: _____

_____

_____

_____

As you can see, one value can produce many goals. If you want another step, you need to figure out which goal means the most to you and which one you want to start with. It can be tempting to change your whole life all at once, but take it one step and one SMARTY goal at a time.

> *You do not rise to the level of your goals. You fall to the level of your systems.*
>
> —James Clear, *Atomic Habits: An Easy & Proven Way to Build Good Habits and Break Bad Ones*

Are You Heading East?

If you're confused about whether a goal you're setting is healthy and in alignment with your value, ask yourself one question: *Are you heading east?* What the heck does that mean? Let me explain: Imagine you're on a road trip with no real destination in mind; you just know what direction you want to go. You look at your compass (your values) and realize they are east. From there on out, every stop you make (aka every goal you set) on that road trip should be heading east, aka working toward living your values. This can be a big problem solver when you're stuck.

Are the goals you're setting and the actions you're taking to meet them sending you east? Asked another way, this simply means: Are my goals taking me in the right direction, toward my values? Whenever you get into a rut, you can ask yourself this simple question to get a better perspective on what you're doing and what you should be doing.

Your Chase Values, Crush Goals Statement

The Chase Values, Crush Goals Statement is what ties all of these ideas together. It's basically a major goal you would like to achieve, detailing how you will achieve it, your time frame, and your big why. Think of it like a contract with your physical AND higher self. Here's an example:

> Beginning in May, I will start training to run a half-marathon, and I will run it by the end of September. Accomplishing this goal will help me get back in shape so that I can run around with my kids. To ensure the success of this goal I'll commit myself to buying appropriate running shoes, joining a local running club and/or hiring a running coach, running at least four times a week, and running a race at least once a month.
>
> I'm chasing this goal because of my nephew. My brother passed away a few years back, and I vowed to be the positive father figure and male role model for my nephew that I never had growing up. I also want to instill the value that physical activity and health is possible at every size. The best way for me to do this is to lead by example while he's young.

Take a few minutes to think about what you want, why you want it. Then write your own Chase Values, Crush Goals Statement.

_____

_____

_____

_____

_____

_____

_____

_____

_____

_____

_____

Use the above as a template if you like. Revisit it when you feel you need a reminder of what you're putting yourself through the running struggle for. Revisit it when you feel amazing and you realize you're actually doing the damn thing.

When you reach that big goal, start over again. Look east. Write. Crush goals. Repeat.

Advanced Goal Crushing: Building Your Action Plan

> *Passion alone can't cut it. For passion to survive it needs structure. A why without how has little probability of success.*
>
> —Simon Sinek, *Start with Why: How Great Leaders Inspire Everyone to Take Action*

Okay! Now you're about to get into some advanced content. If you're feeling like you have enough to chew on, this is a good place to stop. If you want to do a really deep dive into some heavy-duty routine-building stuff, buckle up and get ready for the ride of your life. Because everything is about to change after this section. You've been warned! Let's take a look at what we've put together in this chapter so far.

Compass calibrated with clear, defined values? *Check!*

Destination defined with SMARTY goals? *Check!*

Pre-road checklist with an action plan in place? *Chec—* No! Wait, what?!?!

That's right. Just because you have your values and goals in place doesn't mean that you're necessarily good to go. You need to set up an action plan, too. An action plan, also called a process, is a detailed plan outlining the steps needed to reach a particular goal. Yes, you may have a clear, beautifully written goal, but you also want to have a process describing how you plan to complete that goal, as this will give you a higher chance of success!

When creating action plans for reaching your goals, here are a few questions to think about:

- What steps do you need to take to accomplish the goal?
- What or who can help you complete these steps?
- When do you plan to start each step?
- What is the deadline for completing each step?
- What order should you complete the steps in?

I've included a worksheet below to help you build your first action plan—as well as all your plans after that. Choose the most important goal from your earlier list and list all the possible next steps that could help you reach that goal.

They don't have to be in any particular order yet. Just jot them down under "action steps" in the table below. Once you've identified your action steps, think about what resources you will need to complete each step. Write these under "resources." Next, determine which step you should do first, second, third, and so on. List them in order under "priority." Finally, determine the start dates and deadlines for each step. Once you have your process in place, it's time to get to work executing your plan. Every so often, maybe once a week or once a month, you should monitor, evaluate, and update your processes as needed.

Value:					
SMARTY Goal:					
Action Steps (What do you need to do to reach this goal?)	Resources (Who or what can help you complete this step?)	Priority (Which step comes first? What comes next?)	Start Date (When do you plan to start this step?)	Due Date (By when do you need to complete this step?)	Comments

Rituals and Habits

We began this chapter with the big picture, by addressing values, which are your compass; they define the direction you want your life to go. Then we worked on defining your goals, which are your destinations on this road trip we call life. After we set some goals, we defined the action plan or processes that can help you accomplish those goals. But we're not done yet!

You can start to cross things off your process list, such as buying running shoes, choosing a training plan, or finding a place to run, but you still have to actually start running. And this is where rituals come in. I know what you're thinking: *Martinus! What the heck are you talking about?! What is a ritual and how does it fit into my action plan?* So glad you asked.

A ritual is a sequence of activities; it may involve gestures, words, actions, or objects, and it consists of actions that are performed according to a set sequence. Rituals are not the same as habits, but they can help form habits. Habits are actions like running or brushing your teeth; rituals are a series of actions that support the execution of the main habit. For example, once you start consistently running, it's a habit. Your running rituals might include your pre-run warm-up or the cooldown that you use after your run.

Also, a habit can be done mindlessly, on autopilot, but a ritual should be done with full intention, presence, attention, and mindfulness. If you're a runner, rituals are behaviors that you maintain even when you're not training for a race. They solidify your identity as an athlete. They are actions that reinforce your lifestyle, your mindset, and your general trajectory toward becoming a runner and living as an athlete.

Some of the most successful professional athletes and performers use rituals. For example, before every show, Beyoncé listens to the same playlist, says a prayer with her band, completes a specific set of stretches, sits in her massage chair while getting her hair and makeup done, and spends exactly 1 hour meditating.

Serena Williams bounces the ball exactly five times before her first serve and two times before her second serve. Meb Keflezighi usually eats a bagel or Himbasha (homemade Eritrean bread) with honey before a race. He prepares this breakfast the night before the race and puts it on his nightstand. So if he wakes up in the middle of the night, he can have an early breakfast without even leaving his bed.

I even used rituals while writing this book. Every day, I woke up around five A.M. and ate a quick breakfast while listening to the same playlist of songs before I started writing. This repeated ritual put me in the mindset to write.

Rituals are the key to success; they are what help you establish good habits. Rituals can help focus your mind and calm your nerves during performance. Studies show that practicing rituals before doing sports reduces stress and anxiety and increases mental toughness. Similarly, rituals such as affirmations, specific actions (placing a bagel on your nightstand the night before a race), or even lucky charms have been shown to improve athletic performance and motor dexterity. Rituals give us a sense of control in a world filled with uncertainties. That's why I think habits should always be paired with rituals. Rituals can complement your routines and protect you from bad habits. Rituals help create natural flow in your routines by overcoming barriers that may be blocking you from developing a positive new habit.

Look back at the goals and processes you listed in the worksheets provided earlier in this chapter. Now brainstorm some habits that can help you accomplish those goals and stick to those processes, and list them in the habit tracker below.

Here are some suggested habits to give you some ideas:

- Go running consistently.
- Get 8 hours of sleep a night.
- Drink 64 or more ounces of water each day.
- Cross-train.
- Foam-roll.

Habit Tracker

Use this to track when and whether you engage in your planned habits. List the habits you want to implement in the far-left column and write an X on the days that you completed the habit. (For a PDF version of this habit tracker and other worksheets in this chapter, check out chapter 9 of the Slow AF Run Club Bonus Companion Course at slowafrunclub.com /course.)

Date																															
Habit	1	2	3	4	5	6	7	8	9	10	11	12	13	14	15	16	17	18	19	20	21	22	23	24	25	26	27	28	29	30	31

Defining Rituals

Next, we are going to brainstorm some rituals to support your habits. Some rituals might come naturally, but others are good to think about beforehand.

In the space provided, write down a habit that you would like to create a ritual for.

Example: Go for a run every other day at seven A.M.

_____

_____

_____

Next, list steps or action items that will help you perform this habit.

Example: Lay out my clothes the night before; set a bagel on my nightstand like Meb.

_____

_____

_____

_____

_____

Now, identify a trigger for this ritual.

Example: I'll lay out my clothes after my nightly shower.

_____

_____

_____

_____

_____

Are there any diversions or distractions that typically interrupt your routines? Can you plan ahead for these issues and incorporate, eliminate, or minimize them? Write down how below.

_____

_____

_____

_____

_____

Once you have your ritual mapped out, you can name it. Make it fun and get as creative as you want with this. It's a great way to make it your own.

Example: Badass Pre-running Nighttime Routine

_____

_____

_____

And there you have it. Remember, you can revise the elements of your ritual as needed.

GOAL-SETTING QUESTIONS ASKED BY EVERY BEGINNER, NONTRADITIONAL, SLOW, OR FAT RUNNER

1. How do I not beat myself up when I can't reach a goal? How can I forgive myself when I don't reach a goal?

    First, remember that a goal is only part of the journey, it's not the journey itself. We are all going to have goals that we're dead set on completing—only to fall flat. It wasn't in the cards, and that's okay. The fact that you were going after that goal is reason to celebrate! You tried and you did something that helped you to continue to go east. Zoom out and look at the bigger picture. Did it contribute to your larger value? Yes? Then it's time to celebrate. No? Maybe it's time to look at another goal more in line with your values!

2. How do I adapt/reset when a goal isn't working for me?

Ask yourself: Am I going east? Look at your goal. Does it serve the purpose of your values? If not, drop it, look at your goal list, and start the process again. Simple as that. If yes, think about why the goal isn't working for you anymore. Are you frustrated about the lack of progress? Are you putting in as much work as it requires? Is it something else? It's time to get to the root of the issue. When you're honest with yourself, pivoting to a new goal is easy. You can always come back to it in the future!

3. What does a reasonable running goal look like? I so often dream big, get overwhelmed, and fizzle.

I believe all goals can be reasonable with the right timeline, even big running goals (yes, like a marathon). That is why making SMARTY goals is important. If you want to run a marathon, consider your timeline. If you want to run a marathon next month and you ran a marathon four weeks ago, that's a reasonable goal. However, if you want to run a marathon next month and you've never run a marathon or even trained for one, then that's definitely not reasonable. It's all about context and timeline. Anything is possible with time and dedication!

Now that you know everything you need to become a goal crusher for today, tomorrow, and the years to come, continue reading, because in the next and final chapter, we are talking about finding your people.

CHAPTER 10

(Running) Communities: Finding Your People

Cautionary Tale: Slow Runner Left Behind

When I moved to the San Francisco Bay Area (see chapter 8), I didn't have any friends, I had nobody to go running with, and I didn't even know the good places to run. I figured all those problems could be fixed by finding a running club to join. In the past, I'd had the absolute worst luck finding a run club, but since I was in a new area, I was hopeful to find the crew I'd been looking for.

I went to the internet, did some research, and found a club that seemed promising. It had all the buzzwords I was looking for: *all paces welcome, all ages and abilities welcome, friendly, inclusive.* This sounded like my type of club. I dug further and checked the group's socials and website to find out as much as I could. The story seemed to check out!

Yes! I think I found my people.

I was so excited to run with a new crew and decided to

participate in its beginner 3-miler that following Sunday. (Even though I was not a beginner, over the years I've learned that *beginner* is a code word for slow, but that's another story.)

When the day came, I headed to their meetup spot and introduced myself.

"Hi, I'm Martinus. I'm new to the area, and I'm training for the New York City Marathon." One of the captains scoffed and responded with something along the lines of "Oh, wow, you're training for New York? Shouldn't you try a shorter distance and lose weight first before you try to run a marathon?" That same old fatphobic BS. (Strike one!)

My jaw almost hit the ground. I started to do an about-face to leave. This wasn't the first time that someone had passed judgment on me, and it wouldn't be the last. It still happens all the time, even though it shouldn't. Something kept me from walking away, though. I have been dealing with such attitudes my whole life, so funnily enough, I'm quick on my feet.

"This isn't my first marathon, and quite frankly, my weight is none of your business. I thought this was a friendly and inclusive group?"

"Well, it is," he responded.

"It doesn't seem like it to me."

"Whoa, let's not get started on the wrong foot," someone interjected. "What he was trying to say—"

"I know what he said," I interjected, "and I can infer his meaning. From this side of the conversation, that question wasn't friendly *or* inclusive."

The original captain apologized. At that moment, I should have left, but part of me wanted the arrangement to work out. They inquired about my pace. When I said I could run somewhere around a 13- to 14-minute mile for a 3-miler, they said their slowest pacer ran at 10 minutes per mile.

"You'll have to try your best to keep up with them."

"I thought all paces were welcome," I objected.

"Well, they are, it's just that we never needed anything above a 10-minute-per-mile pace." (Strike two!)

It was clear that all paces were *not* welcome when someone running a pace that wasn't the norm showed up. I knew this was going to be a bad fit for me, and I should have listened to my intuition, but since I was already there, I decided to give it a try. (Folks, let me stop right here and say LISTEN TO YOUR INTUITION. It's usually right. If I had listened, I would have been long gone. But NOOOO, I stayed. Now I'm here, writing this.)

After we warmed up and did drills, we started running. Initially I tried to keep up with the 10-minute pace group, but it just wasn't happening. I was with the pack for all of 7 minutes before I started to drift behind. You know that feeling I talked about in chapter 2 when I was running in between those gazelles in the fitness center? Yeah, I was there again. I fought a losing battle because there was no way in hell that I could keep up.

I stopped running and took a walking break. The pacer did a double take but never stopped running with the pack as he shouted back to me, "Keep up, big man!"

"I'm good!" I yelled back. "I'm going to run intervals."

As the gazelles continued to disappear around a curve on the trail, I kept walking. I shook my head in disappointment and kicked myself for not listening to my gut. I was realizing that the club's description of itself had been too good to be true.

When my walk break was over, I started running again, making my way around the curve in the trail that the gazelles had just disappeared around. I was met with an intersection of another trail, and the gazelles were nowhere in sight. I stood at the intersection, scratching my head, thinking that, like Bugs Bunny, I should've taken that left turn at Albuquerque. Which way did they go? I stood there for another couple of minutes, hoping something would give me an inkling of which direction to take. Another feeling rushed over me, and I shook my head, turned around, and started to make my way back to where we had started.

Unfortunately I got turned around because we had crossed multiple intersections of trails. I was lost, alone, and hadn't found the running crew I was looking for. Damn.

"Hey, do you know where the runners went?" I asked one of the runners who had been in another pace group as he came around from the curve on the left. He was also a person of size, and I'd seen him briefly when I was warming up.

"No, the group left me. I was running back to the parking lot and got turned around."

"They left me, too. I'm going back to the parking lot as well. You can run with me," I said.

"Hey, just to warn you, I run intervals."

"Me, too!" It was such a relief. We ended up having a great conversation about running and eventually exchanged phone numbers so we could meet and do more running together.

When we finally made it back to the parking lot, some of the run club was already back.

I heard, "Hey, big guy, what happened to you?" It was the captain of the 10-minute-mile pace group.

"Y'all left me, and I got lost."

"Oh, well, the route to the run is in the Meetup."

"Nobody told me the route was posted anywhere."

He shrugged his shoulders and walked away. They didn't have to worry about seeing me again. I got in my car and drove home in silence, reflecting on my experience. I was upset at myself for letting this experience go this far. On the other hand, I had found a new trail and potentially a new running buddy. So I guess there was a silver lining to my story.

Does this story sound familiar? Or are you afraid to try a running club because you think that something like this will happen to you? If you answered yes to one of these questions, keep on reading! In spite of this terrible experience, I eventually went on to find a crew of runners who would support me while I was in the San Francisco Bay Area, and it gave me the insight to create the Slow AF Run Club.

While there are some (in fact, probably many) shitty run clubs out there, the tides are turning. Hell, I was just on the cover of *Runner's World* magazine, so you know the tides are turning. Running is becoming more inclusive. I wouldn't rule out running clubs and crews just yet.

In this chapter, we'll discuss the importance and benefits of finding your people. I'll share tips about what to look for with running clubs and crews, explain how to find the right running community for you, and provide some advice for running with others.

The Benefits of a Running Community

I know what you're probably thinking: *Martinus, I don't want to go through the hassle of finding a community. I don't see any benefit to it. Plus, why would I willingly put myself into a situation where I'm gonna be called out, abandoned in the dust of gazelle runners, and left to fend for myself out in the Serengeti?*

Whoa, grasshopper, before you throw the baby out with the bathwater, let me tell you something! I've been through it all. I'm writing this book for you so you can be the best runner you can be. I'm going to get you through this. We're going to help you find your people and it's going to be great!

There are tons of benefits to having a running community. It's so important to be surrounded by like-minded, supportive people, especially true when you're training for an event or race. You may find it tough to get out the door and hit the pavement when you're running by yourself. Even if your intentions are good, the excuses can be many: the weather is dreary, the dog ate your shoelaces, or you're just not feeling it. This is where social support comes in handy—it's the key benefit of joining a running community. While all of this sounds fine and dandy in theory, let's break down how social support works for you when you join a running community.

Encouragement

Have you ever exercised hard and felt like you can't do any more, but when you're about to quit someone says, "You got this. Keep going," and it's just the lift you need to finish the workout? (If you haven't, you will soon.) Yeah, that's encouragement. It can be difficult to keep on moving forward with running when you are alone, but it's much easier when you have other people around who share your goals and encourage you along the way.

When you start to run for the first time, it can be hard. It's unfamiliar territory. Many of the people who I coach second-guess and doubt themselves—a lot. This is where the encouragement from a running community can really help. Having someone to validate your feelings and cheer for you to keep at it is a game changer!

Encouragement can also take the form of having someone to complain to or to help you cope when you don't feel like heading out on that run. For example, when I'm not feeling it, I call my friend, and he generally knows what to say to get me laced up and outside. He will go as far as talking to me throughout my whole run, and depending on the time, he'll go for a run or walk, too, while we are on the phone.

Accountability

Have you ever scheduled a morning run alone, but then hit the snooze button and skipped it? You can't do that with a running buddy!

Accountability creates consistency because there's pressure

coming from outside of you. A running community can provide this important sense of accountability. Runners who have social support are more likely to stick with their running routines than those who don't. When you're in a community and you all are striving toward your respective goals, it's much harder to slack off or skip a run without feeling bad about it or like you're letting the rest of the crew down by not being there. These group expectations can be really helpful in keeping you on track and motivated to reach your goals. Plus, if your running community meets IRL, there's something incredibly satisfying about completing a workout with a group of other people and having someone waiting for you at the end to high-five you.

Basically it's easier to stay motivated when you know there are others counting on you, AND it makes the process more fun. Accountability in running communities can take many forms. The easiest method is finding a partner who wants to start changing their own habits as well. Maybe that person wants to work out more often, too. This means that when one person skips, then both are missing an opportunity to move together. Another option is signing up for races together; there's no better motivation than knowing you have a friend training with you who will run alongside you throughout the race.

Camaraderie

Training for a marathon is long and tough, and you can be out there for hours, weekend after weekend, for months. Sometimes it's fun, and sometimes it sucks. What I can guarantee is that it sucks LESS if you have people to go through it with you, literally beside you. Having people support you at home is helpful, but there's nothing that forges friendships faster than really going through it together. Basically other runners understand like nobody else can.

When we spend time with folks who know what we're going through and understand us, it can make us feel like we belong. Communities give runners the sense of being part of something bigger than themselves. Running can be a solitary and dull sport, but it doesn't have to be. Finding camaraderie and a sense of belonging with people who understand what you are going through and support you—all of this contributes to a runner's well-being and happiness. These feelings are hard to come by anywhere else and are priceless.

When I was training to run the Boston Marathon, I trained with a runner crew in New York City. Before I started training with them, my experience was trash. BUT when I started training with them, running hills in Central Park in the dead heat of summer sucked less. Don't get me wrong, it still sucked. But we suffered together.

Furthermore, training together helps create friendships and bonds between people who might otherwise not know one another. The camaraderie that happens when you do hard things together makes life so much more special and memorable for everyone involved.

Bonus: Research shows that people who exercise in groups gain greater enjoyment from their workouts and feel less fatigued when they're finished. Social support in a team setting can enhance performance during sports and exercise via reductions in physical discomfort and fatigue.

Sharing Resources and Knowledge

Running communities are a great resource for crowdsourcing information on races, training programs, nutrition, and gear. The beauty of being part of a running community is that there's always someone who's been around the block a few times and can help you troubleshoot what you're currently experiencing (exhaustion, soreness, second-guessing yourself), so they can give you advice on how to get past it.

How to Find the Right Running Community for You

Finding the perfect running community can be hard. Think about your needs before you go out and start looking for one, because all communities are not created equal! Are you just seeking social interaction, or would you like to train with other people? Are these social clubs with no training goals or are they more of a competitive environment, focused on group coaching for specific distances, races, or events? What time of day would best suit your schedule—dawn patrol morning runs, runching (running at lunch), hill repeats after work, or nighttime beer runs? What size group are you looking for? A large corporate running entity or a small local club? These are all issues to consider before you start looking for a club. Once you have an idea of what you're looking for, it's time to start searching! Lucky for you, we've got lots of places to look.

> **Phone a friend, family member, or coworker.** We all know someone who is an avid runner. Why not get in touch with that person in your network and ask for recommendations? They may have their thumb on the pulse of the running scene in your area.
>
> **Local running shoe stores** can be another great resource. If you have access to a specialty running shoe store in your area, I would suggest starting there. Most local running stores either have their own running clubs or have running clubs meeting there. This can be a great way to meet other runners in your area, as well as to get advice from experts!
>
> The other cool thing about joining a club that meets at a running shoe store is that you'll get to know when new shoes come out. When I was meeting with this one club out of a running shoe store, I became good friends with the manager, and an employee would call me whenever my favorite shoes came in. One time, I was struggling to find a new shoe when my old shoes changed style and fit (see chapter 3). The manager pulled out every shoe that the store had in my size and let me try them out on the treadmill until I found the right shoe.

Another perk with a running club that's attached to a shoe store is that sometimes members-only special discounts, promotions, and perks are included when you're part of the group. The store can help you get connected to local races, so don't forget to ask about that as well! Keep in mind that if the group doesn't fit your needs, there will likely be others at the same location looking for a team. Many stores have multiple groups going on at once (for example, one that's focused on running and another that has social gatherings). Ask around and see what fits best with your schedule or personal preferences.

Local running clubs are a great option. If you're looking for something more structured, then joining a running club is definitely worth considering. Depending on where you live, it can be super easy to find one online. Just go to your favorite search engine and type in "running clubs [your city here]." You can also find clubs through the Road Runners Club of America website. There are so many running clubs that have a wide range of abilities and paces, so you're sure to find one that fits your needs. And because they are local, you'll be able to meet other runners in your community in person!

Race organizers can be another good resource. If you've been eyeing a specific race, it may be worth reaching out to the race organizer to ask them about running clubs. They may have affiliations with running clubs and crews that partici-pate in their races yearly. They will be more than happy to forward these groups' contact information to you.

You may also want to consider charity race teams. A great way to give back and meet new people is by participating in charity races or on a charity race team. Usually, large races that are hard to get into will have a charity component that allows you to raise money to get a bib for the race. Most of the time, these charities have running clubs and crews attached to them to provide training programs to help runners get race-ready. This kills two birds with one stone. Not only will you feel good about running for a great organization, but you'll also make some new friends along the way!

Social media is another good place to start. Many runners use social media sites to find new friends who run. Individual runners often create groups that you can easily join. This is a great way to find people in your area who share the same interests as you. And because it's online, there's no pressure to show up if you don't feel like it; you can just chat with everyone through the group's message board. Meetup is another great resource that can help you find groups in your area with similar interests, like running.

Virtual clubs like the Slow AF Run Club provide you with all the social support benefits directly from the comfort of your home. Furthermore, you'll have members from a wide range of locations, which is great because if you are traveling for races, you may find someone in the group who is traveling to the same race. The Slow AF Run Club is a great place to meet new people and make friends with runners who share the same goals as you. You can easily ask questions, offer advice, or talk about anything under the sun. It's also great for meeting partners for your training runs. There are other virtual clubs out there, too, but honestly? Yours truly is a little biased on the subject (and you can see why at slowafrunclub.com! #ShamelessPlug).

Finally, if all else fails, **start your own run club.** If you build it, they will come. Despite all the options available, you may still find that your needs are not being met. So start your own community! That's why I created Slow AF Run Club. I couldn't find the right support for myself as a slow, fat, nontraditional runner, so I created my own group. Other great examples of grassroots groups that reach underserved runners are **Black Girls Run, Black Men Run, Latinos Run, and GirlTrek.**

These communities were all started because there was a need waiting to be filled. Still, I would exhaust all other options before starting your own club. It's a lot of work and responsibility to be the person who everyone looks to for direction on their running journey. (Especially when you're just beginning your running journey!)

There are many ways to find a running community, and these are just a few of the most popular options. Do some research and see what works best for you, but remember, there's no wrong way to do this! The important thing is that you're getting out there and meeting new people. Who knows? You may even make some lifelong friends along the way!

What to Look for in Running Clubs and Crews

Now that you've found some running communities, here are some ways to pare them down to find your perfect fit. We want to avoid you experiencing any cautionary tales of your own!

For starters, reflect on your needs from earlier in this chapter. Get in touch with a group's organizers and ask them about their policies, including whether you need to be a member of the club before joining an event. Ask about membership fees and dues to see if it's worth it for you. Try to find reviews online from other runners who were satisfied with the group or ask to speak to other members of the club. Make sure the group offers what you want regarding time, pace, distance, or meeting frequency. Don't be shy to be up-front about your pace, and do NOT be afraid to ask questions. Lots of them.

Ask how they support runners with a slower pace. Ask them what they do if runners fall behind. Do they leave them, or do they have someone in the back to make sure that no one is running alone? Lastly, when trying out new clubs, don't forget what's important—safety first! Make sure that there are always people around at these events, so it doesn't feel like you're on your own.

And if you start running with a club and find yourself in a bad situation (as I did in the cautionary tale at the beginning of the chapter)? Get the fuck out of there! There's no shame in walking away from a situation where you aren't having any fun. You're not walking away out of weakness, but because the club is not serving your purpose. Running is supposed to be fun! You deserve to have fun! Got it?

Tips for Running with Other People

Ready to make the leap into running with others? That's great! Whether you're running with another person or heading out with a group, here are a couple of quick tips to prepare you for running in a social setting. (Yes, it's different.)

- **Decide on some ground rules.** Who's the leader of this run? Music or no music? Talking or not talking? Discuss the goal of the run. Are we pushing each other? Is it a long, slow run? Intense training run? A social run? Talk about your running pet peeves before you take off; that way you all don't get on one another's nerves.
- **Let slower runners set the pace.** This is pretty self-explanatory. It's important to stay near each other, so adjust accordingly. Don't sprint ahead unless this was agreed upon before the run. If you want to head out with a runner who is faster than you, plan to join the runner for their recovery run, so you can comfortably run together.
- **Don't be afraid to advocate for yourself.** If you need to slow down or take a restroom break, say it.

- **Arrive on time.** If your running buddies are counting on you to meet them for a run, be sure to show up when they expect you to! They have put in the effort to get their workout in, so don't make them wait!

- **Be open to suggestions.** If the person you're running with suggests something different than what you had planned, do it! You can always go back and run your own route another time. (Unless their route is a 10-miler and you have a 3-miler booked in for that day . . .)

- **Be encouraging.** Encouragement is great for everyone, not just people who are new to running with others or have never run before. There's nothing wrong with giving encouragement when your partner hits a new milestone in their training, either—that's what friends are for!

COMMUNITY QUESTIONS ASKED BY EVERY BEGINNER, NONTRADITIONAL, SLOW, OR FAT RUNNER

1. **What do I do if there are no folks close to me?**

   Don't be discouraged. There are so many different running clubs out there. Different clubs each have their own personality and ethos. So it may take a while to find an IRL club to suit you. In the meantime, if you can't find one to fit your style, try joining a virtual running club like the Slow AF Run Club. That way you can still have some community until you find some folks locally who you can run with.

2. **Should I train to get faster to keep up with the group?**

   No. If the group doesn't have someone at your pace to run with or isn't at least willing to accommodate your pace, then that group isn't the group for you.

3. Should I pack anything different for a group run versus running alone?

I wouldn't for the first couple of times. I'm all about saving
myself just in case. However, once you start to get comfortable
with them, you can decide what to bring and not bring.

4. How do I overcome the fear of running with others and the
shame of not being able to keep up?

You're just going to have to give it a try. If the group you are
running with is inclusive, they will take care of you and make you
feel comfortable regardless of your pace. #NoRunnerLeftBehind

If you are a slow, fat, or nontraditional runner, you'll likely find out
that the running world can sometimes be elitist. Have patience and
courage and you'll find your people. I've made some amazing friends
from the running clubs I've joined, but it took me putting myself out
there.

It can be scary. Nobody wants an awkward conversation about
weight, speed, or whatever. Sometimes you will have bad experiences,
but don't give up. While some people are stuck in their bigoted beliefs,
the world is definitely changing.

Just remember that you're a runner, too, and you'll find a place to
belong if you keep trying. (Or at least join the Slow AF Run Club! We
are here for all your running needs. Check us out at slowafrunclub
.com or download the Slow AF Run Club app on your Apple or Android
device. #ShamelessPlugAgain)

AFTERWORD

When I began my running journey more than ten years ago, all I wanted was a friendly voice of experience, someone to understand exactly what I was going through. Someone to push back against the stigma and the doubt, put a hand on my shoulder, and tell me I was going in the right direction.

I didn't find that person. I had to learn all my lessons the hard way, and in the words of Jay-Z, Martinus did that, so hopefully you won't have to go through that. It's my hope that by sharing my experiences and hard-earned knowledge, I have become the person that I needed all those years back. Thank you for buying this book. It's my honor to pay the work forward.

I want to leave you with some words that I wished somebody would have told me when I started: **you have everything you need to be a runner.**

Of course you can read more books, watch videos, read message boards, and search social media for more information, but I am here to tell you that right now, right here in this moment, **the only thing you gotta do is take action. One action, a little bit at a time.**

This book is jam-packed with information and it can feel overwhelming, like you're trying to take a sip of water from a fire hydrant.

You don't have to go out and change everything in your life all at once. Just pick one thing that really resonated with you and go out and try it. If it works for you? Perfect, add it to your repertoire. If it doesn't? It's not the end of the world. You tried something new, and now you can try something else. Remember, you're going on a journey to figure out what methods work best for you. The beauty of running lies in the fact that your destiny is always in your own hands. No one can run those miles for you. No one can put one foot in front of the other but you. No one can cross the finish line for you. You and only you are controlling your destiny. **You have everything you need to be a runner.**

Also, I've shared cautionary tales to show you some of the adversities I've faced in my running journey. However, my adversities and your adversities may look different. What will be the same is the way that we overcame adversity. **Doing hard things gives you grit and makes you capable of doing even harder things.** So as you face your own challenges, keep that nugget in mind.

Finally, as you continue your running journey, you're going to encounter other people in the same shoes that you and I were in. It's now your duty to help those people. Be the person I needed, the person you needed, the person they need. You don't have to know everything about running to help. Something like a smile, a wave, or a nod out on the road can be the only thing that stands between someone giving up running for good and staying the course.

Thank you for buying this book. Remember, you've got this! Take it slow at the beginning, slowly ramp up as you find your groove, and give it all you got.

See you at the finish line.

Together in the struggle,
Martinus Evans

SLOW AF RUN CLUB
BONUS COMPANION COURSE

All of the chapters in this book include some sort of exercise, assignment, training plan, or worksheet to help you with your running. To get the most out of this book, you might find it helpful to keep track of all of these things and your progress in an organized way.

Although it's not required, I highly recommend you access the free companion course that I've created for you, which you can find at slowafrunclub.com/course. In this free course, you'll get access to supplemental materials, including PDF downloads and video instructions. The materials in the course are organized to match the chapters and sections of this book, which makes it easy for you to find what you need as you read along.

Visit the following link to get free access to your Slow AF Run Club bonus materials now, and I'll see you inside!

slowafrunclub.com/course

SHOUT-OUTS AND ACKNOWLEDGMENTS

Mic check one, two. Is this thing on? Awwww yeah! What's up, party people, let's put our hands together for making it to this section of the book!

Good morning, good afternoon, good evening to you wherever you are in the world! This is your host with the most, Martinus Evans, and I just want to say thanks for reading! You could have read any other book in the world, but you read mine and I appreciate that.

Let's keep the claps going while I give shout-outs to the people who've helped make this book possible.

Come on, y'all, I know you can do better than that!

First and foremost, I want to shout out to my better half, my wife, my ace, my rock, my ride and thrive, Char, for constantly encouraging me throughout this entire process. You have been there for me since day one. Being married to a runner comes with lots of sacrifices, from missed brunches and listening to me complain about races to late nights, earlier mornings, as well as days and weeks alone while I'm out training or traveling. You handle them all and support me tirelessly. This one's for all the times you picked me up on the side of the road, all the random strangers you talked to while you waited hours for me to finish my races, and all those sacrifices. This book wouldn't be what it is without you. If not for your support and encouragement, I wouldn't have had the strength to get through what I've been through to even write it. Truly, thank you for everything.

Come on!

To Slow AF Run Club's copywriter and my first manuscript editor, Riley Wignall: If there is one person who I've talked to about this book the most, and who has looked at its pages as much as I have, it's you. From all of the thought exercises, arguments, and times that you talked me off the ledge, you've been there with me along this book-writing journey and you deserve a big shout-out as well. Thank you for your merciless editing pen. (You know what I'm talking about.)

Shout-out to all my test readers: Alyssa Gail Tolentino; Leroy Kelley; Brooke Hardison; Jamie Hunt; Jetaun Pope; Bethany Steuer; Crystal Mastrianni; Ailton Coleman; Cheryl Bell; Kanoa Greene; Julie Ross; Tamara Evans; Jennifer Cannon; Nikki Massie; Jarelle Parker; my podcast partner in crime, Latoya Snell; and last but certainly not least, Mirna Valerio. Thank you all. The feedback that you provided me helped me turn a good book into a great book.

A big shout-out to the members of the best community for slow runners and walkers on the internet, the Slow AF Run Club! Every time I asked for feedback on a topic, you were all in, ready and willing to share your knowledge as well as your needs and wants for this book. I can't thank you all enough.

To Gina Bianchini and the team from Mighty Networks, the all-in-one community software platform, for sponsoring the Slow AF Run Club app. Thank you for all of your knowledge and support throughout the process of creating the Slow AF Run Club. I'm completely honored to have you in my corner.

I want to give a special thanks to the world's greatest mindset coach, Ameerah Omar, for your contribution on chapter 1.

Shout-out to my literary agent, Sharon Bowers at Folio Literary Management. As well as the Avery/Penguin Random House team, more specifically Lucia Watson, Suzy Swartz, Sally Knapp, Nancy Inglis, Lorie Pagnozzi, Patrice Sheridan, Tom Whatley, Lisa D'Agostino, Yunyi Zhang, Anne Kosmoski, Abby Stubenhofer, Farin Schlussel, Megan Newman, Lindsay Gordon, Casey Maloney, and everyone else who helped make this book possible.

A big thanks to Jessie Zapo, Arjun Saraswat, Becky Gough, Jennifer Thomas, Andre Doxey, Vicky Free, and Barbara Birke.

Shout-outs to my mom, Ora; my sister; Shirley; Mabel aka Clearance Puppy; Charlien and Tyrone Thurmand; Brandy'e Grant; Brandon Jefferson; Tracey and Anthony Moore; Stephanie Onyekwere; Nichol Grady; Julianne Jahr; Danielle Fell; Tyler Austrie; Marcela Pinheiro; and anybody else who gave me words of encouragement while writing this book.

I also want to shout out to the doctor who had the audacity to call me fat, laughed at me, and told me that I was going to die. I still think that you're a fucking dick and an asshole for saying what you said to me. I wish I could remember your name because I would send you this book. I hope that you either improved your bedside manner or aren't practicing medicine anymore, because you sucked as a doctor.

To everyone else who I missed, I just want to say thank you. If you were expecting to see your name and it's not here, thank you as well. You know my heart.

Once again, thank you to everyone who has bought and read this book. You have helped make my dreams into reality. I can't wait to see what we do together next.

NOTES

CHAPTER 3. SHIFTING TO HIGH GEAR (AKA RUNNING DRIP)

49. **63 to 72 percent of the population:** Andrew K. Buldt and Hylton B. Menz, "Incorrectly Fitted Footwear, Foot Pain and Foot Disorders: A Systematic Search and Narrative Review of the Literature," *Journal of Foot and Ankle Research* 11 (2018): 43, https://doi.org/10.1186/s13047-018-0284-z.

CHAPTER 4. CARBS ARE GOOD, F*CK DIETS, AND OTHER RUNNING NUTRITION

65. **Dehydration that causes a loss:** Encyclopedia.com, s.v. "Dehydration," last modified August 13, 2018, https://www.encyclopedia.com/medicine/diseases -and-conditions/pathology/dehydration.

71. **The global dietary supplements market size:** "Report Overview," *Dietary Supplements Market Size, Share & Trends Analysis Report by Ingredient (Vitamins, Minerals), by Form, by Application, by End User, by Distribution Channel, by Region, and Segment Forecasts, 2022–2030*, Grand View Research, accessed September 16, 2022, https://www.grandviewresearch.com/industry-analysis/dietary -supplements-market.

CHAPTER 7. RECOVERY MATTERS

139. **benefits of active recovery include reduced lactic acid buildup:** Olivier Dupuy et al., "An Evidence-Based Approach for Choosing Post-exercise Recovery Techniques to Reduce Markers of Muscle Damage, Soreness, Fatigue, and Inflammation: A Systematic Review with Meta-Analysis." *Frontiers in Physiology* 9 (2018): 403, https://doi.org/10.3389/fphys.2018.00403.

142. **prehab, which involves therapy-based movements:** Amanda Perry and Brittany Marshall, "What Is Prehab?," Ivy Rehab Network, March 21, 2018, https://www.ivyrehab.com/news/what-is-prehab.

CHAPTER 8. CROSS-TRAIN OR DIE! (OR RISK INJURY)

151. **almost half (46 percent) of all recreational runners:** University of Gothenburg, "Major Risk of Injury for Recreational Runners," ScienceDaily, April 12, 2021, https://www.sciencedaily.com/releases/2021/04/210412114832.htm.

151. **you are twice as likely to get a running-related injury:** Pia Desai et al., "Recreational Runners with a History of Injury Are Twice as Likely to Sustain a Running-Related Injury as Runners with No History of Injury: A 1-Year Prospective Cohort Study," *Journal of Orthopaedic & Sports Physical Therapy* 51, no. 3 (2021): 144–50, https://doi.org/10.2519/jospt.2021.9673.

CHAPTER 9. GOALS FOR DAYS (AND MONTHS AND YEARS)

193. **gestures, words, actions, or objects:** Wikipedia, s.v. "Ritual," accessed July 27, 2022, https://en.wikipedia.org/wiki/ritual.

193. **Beyoncé listens to the same playlist:** Elle Alexander, "Beyoncé Reveals Her Preshow Rituals," *Vogue*, May 7, 2013, https://www.vogue.co.uk/article/beyonce-talks-tour-rituals-epic-film.

193. **Meb Keflezighi usually eats a bagel:** Amanda Chan, "What Champion Marathoner Meb Keflezighi Does Before Every Race," Yahoo Health, May 21, 2015, https://www.yahoo.com/lifestyle/mebmebmeb-119448093072.html.

194. **practicing rituals before doing sports reduces stress:** Nicholas M. Hobson, Devin Bonk, and Michael Inzlicht, "Rituals Decrease the Neural Response to Performance Failure," *PeerJ* 5 (2017): e3363, https://doi.org/10.7717/peerj.3363.

194. **rituals such as affirmations, specific actions:** Lysann Damisch, Barbara Stoberock, and Thomas Mussweiler, "Keep Your Fingers Crossed! How Superstition Improves Performance," *Psychological Science* 21, no. 7 (2010): 1014–20, https://doi.org/10.1177/0956797610372631.

CHAPTER 10. (RUNNING) COMMUNITIES: FINDING YOUR PEOPLE

206. **Social support in a team setting:** Arran Davis and Emma Cohen, "The Effects of Social Support on Strenuous Physical Exercise," *Adaptive Human Behavior and Physiology* 4, no. 1 (2018): 171–87, https://doi.org/10.1007/s40750-017-0086-8.

RESOURCES

Angie, Jill. *Not Your Average Runner: Why You're Not Too Fat to Run and the Skinny on How to Start Today.* New York: Morgan James Publishing, 2018.

Bildirici, Lottie. *Running on Veggies: Plant-Powered Recipes for Fueling and Feeling Your Best.* New York: Rodale Books, 2022.

Bingham, John. *Running for Mortals: A Commonsense Plan for Changing Your Life with Running.* New York: Rodale Books, 2007.

Boggs, Meg. *Fitness for Every Body: Strong, Confident, and Empowered at Any Size.* New York: S&S/Simon Element, 2021.

Duckworth, Angela. *Grit: The Power of Passion and Perseverance.* New York: Scribner, 2018.

Galloway, Jeff. *Galloway's Book on Running.* Bolinas, CA: Shelter Publications, 2021.

Galloway, Jeff. *The Run-Walk-Run Method.* Maidenhead, UK: Meyer & Meyer Sport, 2016.

Goggins, David. *Can't Hurt Me: Master Your Mind and Defy the Odds.* Austin: Lioncrest Publishing, 2018.

Green, Louise. *Fitness for Everyone: 50 Exercises for Every Type of Body.* New York: Alpha, 2020.

Grover, Tim S. *Relentless: From Good to Great to Unstoppable.* New York: Scribner, 2014.

Holiday, Ryan. *The Obstacle Is the Way: The Timeless Art of Turning Trials into Triumph.* New York: Portfolio, 2014.

Hutchinson, Alex. *Endure: Mind, Body and the Curiously Elastic Limits of Human Performance.* New York: HarperCollins, 2019.

Marshall, Simon, and Lesley Paterson. *The Brave Athlete: Calm the F*ck Down and Rise to the Occasion.* Boulder, CO: VeloPress, 2017.

Mumford, George. *The Mindful Athlete: Secrets to Pure Performance.* Berkeley, CA: Parallax Press, 2016.

Rye, Tally. *Train Happy: An Intuitive Exercise Plan for Every Body.* New York: Pavilion Books, 2020.

Slow AF Run Club, http://www.slowafrunclub.com.

Summers, Morit. *Big & Bold: Strength Training for the Plus-Size Woman*. Champaign, IL: Human Kinetics, 2021.

Valerio, Mirna. *A Beautiful Work In Progress*. Grand Haven, MI: Grand Harbor Press, 2017.

Verstegen, Mark. *Every Day Is Game Day: Train Like the Pros with a No-Holds-Barred Exercise and Nutrition Plan for Peak Performance*. New York: Avery, 2014.

Willink, Jocko, and Leif Babin. *Extreme Ownership: How U.S. Navy SEALs Lead and Win*. New York: St. Martin's Press, 2017.

INDEX

Note: Italicized page numbers indicate material in tables.

Abbott World Marathon Majors,
    179–80
accountability, 204–5
Achilles tendons, 51
action plans/process, 190–92, *192*
Adidas
    author as ambassador for, x, 16
    running app of, 34
Adidas Runners in New York City, 206
adult-onset runners, 6
advocating for oneself, 211
affirmations, positive, 12–14, 194
air squats, 167
alarms (safety device), 88
allies of minority runners, 90
all-or-nothing mentality, 20, 140
Amazon, shopping for workout
        gear on, 42
American Academy of Sleep
        Medicine, 137
analysis paralysis, 21
anxieties
    around running with others, 213
    managing, 16–18
apps
    for intervals, 32
    for keeping a running journal, 34

shoe mileage tracked by, 53
and treadmill runs, 84
Arbery, Ahmaud, 89
arms
    and good running form, 27
    post-run stretches, 107-9
    Upper/Core Days (cross-training),
        156–65
aspirin, 91, 124
athletic gear
    breaking in, 131
    and the Chafe Monster (*see* lubes to
        prevent chafing)
    checklist of necessary, 37–38
    checklist of nonessential (but nice to
        have), 38
    clothes (*see* workout clothes)
    and dawn/dusk safety
        considerations, 88–89
    designer, 41
    for group runs, 213
    running shoes
        (*see* shoes for running)
    for various run lengths,
        90–92
athletic stance, 104, 156
Atomic Habits (Clear), 188

baby/body wipes, 91, 124
balls for rolling out tight muscles, 143
bamboo, workout clothes made of, 40
bandages, 91, 124
base-building plan, *94–95*
beginner runners
 beginning of your running story, 24–25
 breathing, 29–31
 first run, 32–33
 intervals, 31–32
 keeping a running journal, 33, 34
 pacing, 27–29, 33–34
 rate of perceived exertion, *30–31*, 31
 running form, 25–27, 33
beliefs about running, identifying, 8
belly breathing (diaphragmatic breathing), 29–30
belonging, sense of, 205–6
benefits of running, xii
bent-over rows, 159
Beyoncé, 193
bicep curls, standing, 157–58
bicycling, 139, 151
bird dog (exercise), 161–62
Black Girls Run (club), 210
Black Men Run (club), 210
Black runners, safety considerations for, 89–90
Body Glide lube, 43
body positivity/acceptance
 cultural shift toward, xi
 and plus-size activewear, 40
body/baby wipes, 91, 124
Bolt, Usain, 26
books about running, xi, 225–26
Boston Marathon, 117, 152, 206
breathing
 belly breathing, 29–30
 chest breathing, 29
 and chin placement, 26
 4-7-8 breathing exercise, 138, 138*n*
 and getting started with running, 29–31
 and the lean, 26

 and pacing, 28–29
 through nose vs. mouth, 30
 video demonstrating, 33
brightly colored running gear, 81, 89
butterfly stretch, 109
butt kicks, 105

calisthenics, 151
calorie requirements, calculation for, 68–69
calves
 calf raises, 168–69
 standing calf stretch, 107
camaraderie in running communities, 205–6
carbohydrates
 and carb loading, 75, 122–23
 and complementary proteins, 62–63
 complex carbs, 60, 66
 energy from, 59, 64, 74
 importance of, 74
 and post-run fueling, 70
 and pre-run fueling, 66, 74
 and recovery, 74
 simple carbs, 60–61, 66
cardio cross-training, 151
cell phones, 90, 124
Centers for Disease Control and Prevention (CDC), 137
chafing and the Chafe Monster
 author's first experience with, 35–37
 and compression gear, 42
 and cotton clothes, 38, 40
 lubes to prevent, 43–44, 91, 124
 treating chafed skin, 55
Chamois Butt'r, 44
Char (author's wife), 5, 37, 134, 148
charity race teams, 208–9
"Chase Values, Crush Goals" statement, 189–90
chest breathing, 29
chest press, dumbbell, 162–63
chest tilt, 25–26
chin placement, 26
clamshell (exercise), 165–66
Clear, James, 188

clothing. *See* workout clothes
coconut oil, 43
colors, running gear in bright, 81, 89
companion course, 217
comparison, avoiding, 21, 25
competitiveness, 20, 21
compression gear
   benefits of, 42–43
   compression boots, 136, 143, 145
   and post-race recovery, 145
confidence, 8, 11
consistency
   and accountability, 204–5
   and flexibility in training plans, 111
   making a habit of running, 194
   while getting started with running,
      29, 92, 93
conversation pace (Sexy Pace), 28–29, 34
cooling down, 106–9
   author's routine for, 106
   and lactic acid, 106
   stretching during, 107–9
   walking, 32
cotton clothing, 38, 40
course time limits/cutoff times
   and course types, 117, 118
   and elitism in running, 116
   and picking races to run, 115, 131
   and walker-friendly races, 119
credit cards, carrying, 90
critics and hecklers, responding
   to, 34, 80
cross-arm stretch, 108
cross-training, 147–77
   benefits of, 150
   cardio, 151
   definition of, 150
   eight-week schedule for, *155–56*
   focusing on weaknesses with, 153
   frequency of, 152–53, 176–77
   guidelines for circuit training,
      153–54, 156
   habits for, 194
   importance of, 149–50, 176
   and injury prevention, 151
   Leg Day Circuit A, 165–69

Leg Day Circuit B, 169–73
   and overtraining, 176
   between races, 130
   and recovery, 152, 154
   on rest days, 177
   running on same day as, 177
   strength training, 151
   Upper/Core Day Circuit A, 156–61
   Upper/Core Day Circuit B, 161–65
   while injured, 101n
cupping, 143–44
cycling, 139, 151

Daniels, Jack (running coach), 135
dawn/dusk, running during, 87–89
dead bug (exercise), 159–60
dead butt syndrome, 149
deadlifts, 168, 171
defecating prior to race starts, 124
delayed onset muscle soreness
   (DOMS), 174
delusional self-belief, 15–16
depression/blues after a race, 129–30
DFL (dead fucking last),
   coming in, x, 127
diaphragmatic/belly breathing, 29–30
diet culture, 72, 75, 92
disabilities, runners with, 6
discomfort. *See* pain and discomfort
distance of runs
   and beginner runners, 29
   measured in time rather
      than miles, 35n
   training for distance, 110
distractions, 196–97
DNF (did not finish), 127
DNS (did not start), 127
doctors
   author's experiences with, ix–x, 16,
      22, 142, 180–81
   exams and blood work from, 142
   fatphobia of, ix–x, 22n
   unsolicited lectures from, 22
dogs, running with, 89
doing hard things, 21, 216
donkey kicks (exercise), 170

Douglass, Frederick, 24
down-and-back courses for races, 117
dumbbells
    chest presses, 162–63
    Romanian deadlifts, 171
    shoulder presses, 164
    side raises, 163–64
dynamic stretching, 102

earbuds or headphones, 80, 87–88, 90
elbows and good running form, 27
electrolytes, 70, 91. *See also* water and
    hydration
elite athletes
    dropping out of races, 127
    running instruction offered by, xi
elitism in running
    and course time limits, 116
    and finding your community, 213
    and self-reliance on race days, 126
emergency contact information,
    carrying, 90
emotions, 8–9, 12, 129–30, 140
encouragement
    experienced in running
        communities, 204
    offering, to other runners, 212, 216
energy
    from carbohydrates, 59, 64, 74
    from fat, 63–64
energy management
    and pacing, 28, 31
    on race day, 121
entry fees for races, 120
euphoria experienced during runs, 36
exertion, rate of, *30–31*, 31
expectations management, 125–26
expenses related to races, 120
expos at races, 121

failure, perspective on, 11
fat, dietary
    as energy source, 63–64
    and pre-run fueling, 74
    sources of, 64
fatigue
    from overtraining, 176

and social support in a team, 206
fatphobia
    author's experiences with, ix
    of doctors, ix–x, 22*n*
    in running clubs, 200
fear, managing, 16–18
feet
    and compression boots,
        136, 143, 145
    and good running form, 26
    See also shoes for running
fiber
    benefits of, 61
    as carbohydrate, 59–60
    and pre-run fueling, 74
fire hydrants (exercise),
    169–70
first run
    of author, 22–24
    going for your, 32–33, 92
first week as a runner, 92
fitness trackers, 38
Fitspo, 8
5-4-3-2-1 Grounding
    Technique, 19
5K training plan
    base-building plan, *94–95*
    training plan, *95–98*
foam rolling
    habits for, 194
    as recovery exercise, 139, 143
food-as-fuel principle, 58. *See also*
    nutrition for runners
Footpath app, 84
forefoot landings, 26
form of runners, 25–27
    assessing, 33
    checklist for, 27
    definition of, 25
    the landing, 26, 33
    the lean, 25–26, 33
forward fold, 108
4-7-8 breathing exercise, 138, 138*n*
four-week base-building plan,
    94–95
friendships with other runners, 206
"fuck the world" attitude, 80

fuel packs
    on race day, 124, 125
    on training runs, 91
funeral exercise for examining
        values, 183

gait analysis (shoe fittings)
    costs associated with, 54
    importance of, 45
    recommended frequency of, 54
    what to expect with, 45–46
Garmin app, 84
gear. *See* athletic gear
getting started with running. *See*
        beginner runners
GirlTrek (club), 210
gloves, 38
glucose, 59
glutes
    dead butt syndrome (gluteal
        amnesia), 149
    glute bridges, 166
    weak glutes, 51
goals, 178–98
    action plans for, 190–92, *192*
    adapting/resetting, 198
    definition of, 182
    and motivation, 180–81
    perspective on failure to reach, 197
    and rituals/habits, 192–97
    SMARTY goals, 185–88, *192*, 198
    and values, 181–82, 187–88
Graston tools, 143
gratitude for your body, 129
growth hormones, 137–38

habits, 192–97
    creating rituals to support, 196–97
    rituals' relationship to, 193, 194
    tracking, 194, *195*
hacky sack stretch, 105
half marathons, 44, 130
hands and good running form, 27
hats, 38
headlamps, 88
headphones or earbuds, 80, 87–88, 90
health care professionals, 141–42, 146

heat-related health risks, 77–79
heckling, 80
heel landings, 26
high knees exercise, 105
hobbies, 140–41
home, proximity of running route
        to, 86
hydration packs, 38, 91, 123–24, 123*n*

ice baths, 143
identification, carrying, 89, 90
identity as a runner and athlete,
        9, 24, 193
Imodium chewables, 91, 123
imposter syndrome, 21, 80
inclusivity in running world, 116, 200,
        203, 213
injuries
    and cross-training, 151
    and doing too much, too soon, 111
    high rates of, among runners,
        151, 176
    and missing runs/workouts, 101*n*
    from overtraining, 134–35
    and pain management, 173–76
    and recovering between races, 130,
        135, 146
    responding to, 175–76
    and running form, 25
    from shoes, 44, 51
    and spatial awareness, 175
    and strength training, 151
    training after, 147–48
inner critics, 14–15
insecurity, struggling with, 80
internet
    shopping for shoes online, 48–52
    shopping for workout gear online, 42
intervals
    apps for running, 32
    paces for, 28
    run/walk, 31–32
intuition, listening to, 201

Jordan, Michael, 20
journals, tracking running in, 33, 34,
        109–10

judgments
    author's experiences with, 200
    identifying, 8
    running as a means of conquering, 5
jumping ability, impact of compression
        clothing on, 42

kang squats, 104–5
Keflezighi, Meb, 193
keys, running belts for securing, 38
Kipchoge, Eliud, 15
knowledge, sharing, 206

lactic acid, 106, 139
landings (foot strikes), 26, 33
The Last Dance (documentary), 19–20
lateral lunges, 104, 170–71
Latinos Run (club), 210
lean, 25–26, 33
LED light vest, 38
leggings for running, 37, 38
legs
    and good running form, 26
    Leg Days (cross-training), 165–73
    post-run stretches, 107–9
    pre-run stretches, 104–6
    single-leg Romanian deadlifts, 168
lethargy, 176
LGBTQ+ runners, 6
locations for running, 79–84
    and choosing a route, 84–86
    and dealing with hecklers, 80
    indoor tracks, 84
    and mapping your routes, 84–86
    outdoor tracks, 81–82
    streets and sidewalks, 81
    trail running, 82
    treadmills, 83–84
long runs
    and access to water on running
        routes, 85
    gear to bring on, 91–92, 123
    pre-run fueling for, 66, 123
loop courses for races, 116–17
lotteries for marathon participation,
        178–79

lubes to prevent chafing
    application of, 44
    carrying on training runs, 91
    options for, 43–44
    and race day, 124
    in stick form, 44
lunges
    lateral, 104, 170–71
    runner's, 108–9
    walking, 167–68
Lycra workout clothes, 39

Mace, carrying, 89
MapMyRun app, 34, 84
maps
    of races, 124
    of training routes, 84–86
marathons
    author's determination to
        run, ix–x, 22
    author's first, 1–5
    completed by author, 16
    lotteries for, 178–79
    and lubes to prevent chafing, 44
    and recovering between races, 130
    and SAG wagons, 2–5
    See also specific races, including New
        York City Marathon
Marshalls, shopping for workout gear
        at, 42
massage balls, 143
massage guns, 143
massages and massage therapists, 142
measurements, taking your, 41, 42
Meetup, 209
Megababe, 44
menstruation and period-proof
        gear, 38
mental health, 129–30, 140
mental toughness, 11
midfoot landings, 26
"miles ran," 35n
mindfulness, 18–19, 102
mindset
    and all-or-nothing mentality, 20, 140
    and analysis paralysis, 21

and author's first marathon, 1–5
and bad weather, 21
and comparison, 21
dealing with fear, 16–18
and finding an enemy, 19–20
"fuck the world" attitude, 80
importance of, 5–6
and imposter syndrome, 21, 80
and mindfulness, 18–19, 102
and positive affirmations, 12–14
and practicing delusional self-belief,
    15–16
and recovery, 140–41
and self-perceptions, 7–9
and self-reliance, 9–11, 125–27
and self-talk, 14–15
and success in running, 6
missing runs/workouts, 101, 111,
    173–74
mobile phones, 90, 124
money, carrying, 90, 124
Monistat Care Chafing Relief Powder
    Gel, 43
morning runs, 80
motivation, 180–81, 205
mouth breathing, 30
muscles
    and active recovery days, 139
    building strength in, 62, 63, 151
    and fat consumption, 63
    and fatigue, 42
    and lactic acid, 106, 139
    and protein consumption, 62
    and recovering between races, 136
    and recovery tools, 143
music, listening to, 80, 87–88

natural technical fibers, 40
negativity
    and changing your perceptions, 9,
        11–12
    naming your inner critic, 14–15
    of others, 20, 21
    and overcoming all-or-nothing
        mindset, 20
    and self-talk, 14

neutral pronation, 48, 50, 50
New York City Marathon
    author's experience with, 179
    lotteries for, 179–80
    point-to-point course of, 117
    reactions to author's ambitions to
        run, 200
    size of, 179
    training for, 147–49
nontraditional runners
    definition of, 6
    and self-perceptions, 8
    and self-reliance on race days,
        125–27
    as underserved in running
        community, xi
nose breathing, 30
"No Struggle, No Progress" motto, 24
nutrition for runners, 56–76
    avoiding new foods on race days,
        69–70
    calculation for calorie requirements,
        68–69
    carbs (see carbohydrates)
    fats, 63–64
    and food-as-fuel principle, 58
    foods to avoid before running, 67
    and hitting the wall, 56–57, 58
    importance of, 58
    post-run fueling, 70–71, 73
    pre-run fueling, 66–67, 72–73, 74
    proteins (see protein)
    and recovery, 74–75, 138
    on-the-run fueling, 67–70, 73
    sample day of, 72–73
    supplements, 71, 72–73, 74, 75
    water consumption, 64–65
    and working with a nutritionist,
        58, 76
nutritionists, working with,
    58, 76
nylon workout clothes, 39

odor removal from clothing, 54
outdoors, running in, 80–82
overhead triceps stretch, 108

overpronation, 48, 50, *50*
oxygen, 30

pacing
    for beginner runners, 27–29, 33–34
    and energy management, 28, 31
    and rate of perceived exertion, 31
    for recovery, 28, *30*
    and running clubs, 200–201, 210, 211
    tracking, 33–34
Packer, Randall K., 65
pain and discomfort
    and carrying pain relievers on runs,
        91, 124
    delayed onset muscle soreness, 174
    and knowing when to not run,
        173–74
    pain management, 173–76
    and rate of perceived exertion,
        30–31, 31
    and social support in a team, 206
    soreness compared to, 174, *175*
pants for running, 37, 38
pasta, 75
patience, importance of, 92
people of color
    as nontraditional runners, 6
    safety considerations for, 89–90
Pepto Bismol chewables, 91, 123
perceptions, changing, 11–20
    dealing with fear, 16–18
    and finding an enemy, 19–20
    maintaining positive or neutral
        perspectives, 11–12
    and mindfulness, 18–19
    and positive affirmations, 12–14
    and practicing delusional self-belief,
        15–16
    and self-talk, 14–15
performance, social support's ability to
    enhance, 206
period-proof shorts/leggings, 38
personal identification, carrying,
    89, 90
Phelps, Michael, 143
photographers at races, 125

physical therapists, 142, 148–49
plank (exercise), 160–61
plant proteins, 63
plus-size activewear, 40–44
pocketknives, carrying, 89
point-to-point courses for races,
    117–18
polyester workout clothes, 39
polypropylene workout clothes, 39
pooping before races, 124
Porta-Potties
    access to, 85
    conditions of, on race days, 124, 126
positivity
    choosing, 11–12
    positive affirmations, 12–14
preconceived ideas, identifying, 8
present moment, focusing on, 11,
    18–19
protein
    complete vs. incomplete, 62–63
    importance of, 61–62
    plant proteins, 63
    and post-run fueling, 70
    and pre-run fueling, 66, 74
    and recovery, 74
    sources of, 62
push-ups, 157

quad stretch, standing, 105, 107–8
quick feet exercise, 106

race days
    author's first 5K, 112–14
    avoiding anything new on, 54–55,
        69–70, 122, 131
    breaking in new gear before, 131
    carb loading prior to, 75, 122–23
    choosing races (*see* races, criteria for
        picking)
    day(s) leading up to, 121–23
    distances run prior to, 132
    dropping out of races, 127, 132
    and energy management, 121
    and expos, 121
    and finish-line bottlenecks, 128

fuel/hydration strategies for,
    122–23, 125
  gear to bring on, 123–24
  pacing on, 124–25
  pooping before the race, 124
  post-race depression/blues, 129–30
  post-race rituals/traditions,
    128–29, 145
  preparing for non-inclusive
    experiences on, 126
  and race photographers, 125
  self-reliance on, 125–27
  and staying calm, 121–22, 124–25
  See also recovery
race directors/organizers
  and finding a running club, 208
  and questions about course time
    limits, 115
  sharing race experiences with, 127
  unprepared for slower runners, x
race medals
  and course time limits, 115
  getting, after the race, 128
  and picking races to run, 119–20
  and slow runners, 126
races, criteria for picking, 114–21
  course time limits/cutoff times,
    115–16, 131
  course types/configurations, 116–18
  entry/travel fees, 120
  location of race, 131–32
  and recovering between races, 130
  reviews of races, 120–21
  rolling starts vs. wave starts, 118
  small vs. large races, 118–19
  start times, 120
  time of year, 119
  virtual races, 132
  walker-friendly races, 119
race shirts, 126
rate of perceived exertion (RPE),
    30–31, 31
reasons to start running, 34
recovery, 133–46
  active (shakeout), 138–39
  allowing adequate time for, 130

of author, after car accident, 133–35
  and compression gear, 42, 136,
    143, 145
  and cross-training, 152, 154
  and flexibility in training plans, 153
  food choices for, 74–75
  and health care professionals,
    141–42, 146
  and hustle culture/mindset, 136, 146
  importance of, 135–36
  and losing fitness, 146
  mindset, 140–41
  and muscle repair, 136
  pacing for, 28, 30
  passive, 136–38
  and risk of injury, 130, 135, 146
  routine for, 144–45
  tools/methods used in, 142–44
reflective running gear, 81, 88
resistance training, 139
resources, sharing, 206
rest days
  and active recovery, 138–39
  cross-training on, 153, 177
  and losing fitness, 146
  in training plans, 94–101
  See also recovery
restrooms, access to, 85
reviews of races, 120–21
rituals
  defining, 196–97
  giving priority to, 127
  power of, 192–97
Road Runners Club of America, 208
rolling starts vs. wave starts, 118
Romanian dumbbell deadlifts, 171
routes, considerations for choosing,
    84–86
rows, upright, 164–65
run interval speed, 93
run interval time/distance, 93
Runkeeper app, 34
runner's high, 36
runner's lunge, 108–9
Runner's World, author on cover of, x,
    16, 203

running, definition of, 7
running belts, 38
running clubs and communities
    affiliated with shoe stores, 48, 207–8
    and anxiety of running with
        others, 213
    author's experiences with, 199–202
    benefits of, 203–6
    elitism in, 213
    fatphobic attitudes in, 200
    fees and dues of, 210
    finding a good fit, 206–10
    gear to bring on runs with, 213
    leaving, 211
    non-inclusive, 199–202
    pacing in, 200–201, 210, 211
    speed workouts of, 82
    starting your own, 209–10
    tips for running with other people,
        211–12
    training in order to keep up
        with, 212
    what to look for in, 210–11
running while Black, 89–90
run/walk intervals
    for beginner runners, 31–32
    and safety at races, 125
    and sliders of running, 93–94

safety
    of Black runners, 89–90
    and choosing a route, 86
    and emergency contact
        information, 90
    and headphones, 87–88
    and heat-related health risks,
        77–79
    and personal identification, 89, 90
    and reflective/brightly colored gear,
        81, 88, 89
    and running against traffic, 81, 89
    and run/walk intervals, 125
    and sharing your plans with
        others, 88
    and situational awareness, 87–88
    and visibility, 86, 87–88

and white allies of runners in racial
    minorities, 90
SAG wagons, 2–5
salt tablets, 91, 124
San Francisco Bay Area, 199–202, 203
scenery while running, 86
scholarship entries for races, 120
self-acceptance, 11
self-belief, delusional, 15–16
self-doubt, 204
self-perceptions, 7–9
self-reliance
    embracing mentality of, 9–11
    on race days, 125–27
self-talk, 14–15
"Send Me, I'll Go" (Watkins), 9–11
senior runners, 6
Sexy Pace (conversation pace), 28–29, 34
shade trees on running routes, 85
shaming of slow runners, 116
shin splints, 26
shirts for running, 38
shoes for running, 44–53
    assessing the fit and feel of, 47
    and avoiding new shoes on
        race days, 131
    barefoot, 51
    breaking in, 54–55, 131
    buying multiple pairs of, 52
    buying online, 48–52
    buying your first pair, 44–52
    and checklist of necessary gear, 38
    cushioning in, 51
    and gait analysis, 45–46
    importance of, 44, 53–54
    injuries from, 44, 51
    for under/over- or neutral pronation,
        48, 50, 50
    retiring/replacing, 53, 54
    reviews of, 52
    for road running, 50–51
    shopping tips for, 47–48
    sizes of, 49–50
    and socks, 48
    tracking miles on, 53
    for trail running, 50–51

shoe stores
advantages of shopping at, 48
gait analysis provided by, 45–46
return policies at, 46, 52
running clubs of, 48, 207–8
short runs
gear to bring on, 90–91, 123
pre-run fueling for, 66, 122–23
shorts for running, 37, 38
shoulders
dumbbell shoulder presses, 164
and good running form, 27
side raises, dumbbell, 163–64
Sinek, Simon, 190
single-leg Romanian deadlifts, 168
situational awareness while running, 87–88
sleep, 137–38, 194
sliders of running, 93
Slow AF Run Club
establishment of, x, 16, 203
sharing race experiences with, 127
turtle mascot of, 89
virtual races held by, 132
as virtual running community, 212, 213
slow runners
and self-reliance on race days, 125–27
shaming of, 116
small races, 118–19
SMARTY goals, 185–88, *192*, 198
social media, finding running buddies on, 209
socks, 38, 48
soreness after running, 139, 174, *175*
Spandex workout clothes, 39
spatial awareness, 175
speed
and getting started with running, 29
as low priority, 28
workouts/training for, 82, 82*n*, 110
See also pacing
sports bras, 38, 40–41, 69
sports therapists, 130
sports watches, 32, 38, 70, 84, 125

squats
air squats, 167
kang squats, 104–5
sumo squats, 171–72
Squirrel's Nut Butter, 43
standing biceps curls, 157–58
standing calf stretch, 107
standing quad stretch, 105, 107–8
starches, 59
start times for races, 120
Start with Why (Sinek), 190
static stretching, 102–3
stiffness, 174
strains, 42
Strava app, 34, 84
streets and sidewalks, 81, 89
strength training, 151, 177. *See also* cross-training
stretching
for cooling down, 107–9
dynamic vs. static, 102–3
and lactic acid, 106
for warming up, 104–6
stride length, 26
strobe lights, 88
sugar, 59
summertime
and access to water on running routes, 85
and heat-related health risks, 77–79
and picking races to run, 119
and trees/shade on routes, 85
sumo squats, 171–72
sunglasses, 38
sunlight, 85
sunscreen, 38
superman (exercise), 162
supplements
in author's pre-run breakfast, 72–73
determining need for, 71, 74, 75
and diet culture, 75
industry behind, 71
support received in running communities, 204, 206
surroundings, awareness of, 175

swag as criteria for picking races, 119–20
sweat-loss method of assessing hydration, 71–72
swimming, 139, 151
synthetic technical fibers, 39

talking while running, *30–31*
tape measures, 41, 42
technical fabrics, 39–40
tempo pace, 28, *30*
10K training plan
  base-building, *94–95*
  training plan, *98–101*
tense-and-release mindfulness exercise, 18–19
TENS machines, 143
tensor fasciae latae (TFL) stretch, 108
testosterone, 137
Thanksgiving turkey trots, 120
therapists, seeking help from, 129–30, 140, 146
thirst, 70. *See also* water and hydration
tightness after running, 139
"time ran," 35*n*
TJ Maxx, shopping for workout gear at, 42
toe swipes stretch, 105
Tokyo Olympics (2021), dropout rate in marathon, 127
total duration/distance of run, 93
tracking training in running journals, 33, 34, 109–10
tracks
  advantages of running on, 81–82
  and feelings of insecurity, 80
  and speed workouts, 82
  standard measurements of, 82
traffic
  and beginner runners, 81
  and choosing a route, 86
  running against, 81, 89
trail running, 50–51, 82
training plans
  after your first month, 93–94

after your first three months, 94
and distances run prior to races, 132
eight-week schedule for cross-training, *155–56*
first run, 92
first week as a runner, 92
flexibility in, 111, 152–53, *152*
four-week base-building plan, *94–95*
and missing runs/workouts, 101, 111
and sliders of running, 93
twelve-week 5K plan, *95–98*
twelve-week 10K plan, *98–101*
training runs and rate of perceived exertion, *30–31*
travel expenses, 120
traveling pharmacy, 91, 123–24
treadmills, 83–84
trees and shade on routes, 85
triceps
  triceps kickbacks, 158–59
  triceps stretch, 108
twelve-week 5K plan, *95–98*
twelve-week 10K plan, *98–101*

underpronation/supination, 48, 50, *50*
upright rows, 164–65

values
  "Chase Values, Crush Goals" statement, 189–90
  definition of, 181
  determining, 182–85
  goals' relationship with, 181–82, 187–88
vinegar for odor removal, 54
virtual races, 132
virtual running clubs, 209, 212. *See also* Slow AF Run Club
visibility
  of runners, 87–88
  on running routes, 86
visualization exercises, 102

walking
  as recovery exercise, 139
  and running form, 27
  walker-friendly races, 119
  walk interval speed, 93
  walk interval time/distance, 93
walking lunges, 167–68
wall, hitting the, 56–57, 58
wall sit, 172
Walmart, shopping for workout
  gear at, 41
war analogy for running, 28
warming up, 101–6
  author's routine for, 103
  mental warmup, 102
  stretching, 102, 104–6
watches for runners, 38, 70, 84
water and hydration
  access to, on running routes, 85
  after running, 71, 107
  and electrolytes, 70, 91
  habits for, 194
  hydration vests/packs, 38, 91,
    123–24, 123n
  importance of, 64–65
  on longer runs/races, 91–92, 123–24
  overhydration (hyponatremia), 70
  prior to running, 67
  on race day, 122–23, 124, 125
  during running, 70, 75
  on short runs/races, 90–91
  and sport drinks, 65, 69, 70, 71, 72,
    73, 75, 91
  sweat-loss method of assessing,
    71–72
  and thirst, 70

water bottles, 38
wave starts vs. rolling starts, 118
weather, unpleasant, 21
weight loss, x, xii
wellness, cultural shift toward, xi
where to run. *See* locations for
  running
whistles, carrying, 88
white allies of runners in racial
  minorities, 90
"white people sports," x
will, conquering, 5
Williams, Serena, 193
wool workout clothes, 40
workout clothes
  and the Chafe Monster,
    35–37, 38, 42
  compression gear, 42–43
  in cotton fabrics, 38
  designer, 41
  gloves, 38
  hats, 38
  for larger bodies, 40–44
  and odor removal, 54
  reflective/bright colored, 81, 88, 89
  shirts, 38
  shorts and pants/leggings, 37, 38
  socks, 38, 48
  sports bras, 38, 40–41, 69
  and taking your measurements, 41
  in technical fabrics, 37–38,
    39–40
  See also shoes for running
World Major races, 179–80

yoga, 139, 151

ABOUT THE AUTHOR

Martinus Evans has run more than eight marathons since his doctor told him to "lose weight or die" in July 2012. Since then, he's also coached hundreds of runners and been featured in *The New York Times*, *Men's Health*, *Well+Good*, *The Wall Street Journal*, *New York Post*, LADbible, *HuffPost*, *Magnolia*, and *U.S. News & World Report* and on the cover of *Runner's World*.

To top it off, he's got degrees like a thermometer. He holds a BS in exercise science from Central Michigan University and an MS in health promotion sciences, a graduate certificate in health promotion and health education, and an MA in digital media and design from the University of Connecticut.

When he's not running races around the world, Evans enjoys speaking passionately about issues related to size inclusivity, mindset, DEI, and mental health. He also enjoys playing fetch with his rescue dog, Mabel.